How to Use the Repertory

How To Use The Repertory

with

A Practical Analysis of Forty Homeopathic Remedies

BY

GLEN IRVING BIDWELL, M. D.,

Member American Institute of Homœopathy; New York State
Homœopathic Society; The Society of Homœopathicians;
Monroe County Homœopathic Society; etc.

PHILADELPHIA
BOERICKE & TAFEL
1915

To much of the material, in this little book, I am indebted to
Organon and Chronic Diseases of Hahnemann.   To the
writings and books of Dr. James Tyler Kent.   To the
writings of Doctors A. H. Grimmer, Julia Loos,
Margaret Tyler and R. G. Miller.   To these
physicians as well as all others who are
trying to practice our art and to all
those who are seeking to understand our principles this
book is dedicated.

INTRODUCTION

The degree of vitality Homœopathy enjoys
in any given period will always be indexed by
the methods of its disciples and exponents, not
merely by the soundness of their teaching, but
especially by the thoroughness and accuracy of
their practice. I know of no better gauge of
this vitality than the interest shown in repertory
work, for the repertory is our chief instrument
of precision. True, some men do some good
work without the repertory, but they also do
poor work, more than they would do with it.
A self-made artisan may be a very useful man
although ignorant of the theory and most advanced methods obtaining in his line of work,
but he can never measure up to the man whom
education and thoroughness of method has made
an expert. No such thing as infallibility in prescribing will ever be attained, but he who uses his
repertory faithfully and intelligently—and no
one can do that without equal faithfulness and
intelligence in his study of the Materia Medica—
will inevitably reap his reward, in results and in
that peace of mind that comes only with an ap-
proving conscience. It is encouraging, there-

fore, to realize that there are some who desire to follow the better way,—that there is some demand for such works as this of Dr. Bidwell's, excellently qualified as it is to initiate into effective use of repertory methods; it seems to show that beneath the ashes and debris heaped up by ultra-scientific but essentially chaotic Modern Medicine, burn here and there the embers of a love for therapeutic Truth, which are destined to burst forth at last into a steady, spreading flame that shall bring much good to the children of men.

JAMES TYLER KENT.

PREFACE

The call from the members of our school for an index of the symptoms of our materia medica has been insistent ever since the first edition of the *Materia Medica Pura.* This call has resulted in the publishing of several repertories, from the earliest ones, which covered the few remedies then proven to the last edition of Kent, which is an index to all the remedies proven homœopathically or confirmed clinically to the present time.

When members of our school turn to this vast work for assistance they are confronted with a maze of material, which, to the uninitiated, is more confusing than the materia medica.

It is to help the members of our school who are desirous of mastering and using the repertory that this little work is presented. The repertory, the arrangement and use of which I try to make clear and from which the examples are given, is that of Kent (Second Edition), as this is the only unabridged work we have and the one that is most simple and satisfying to use. The general plan of the repertory work here laid down can be used equally well with any other repertory, the only change needed being that you must master the arrangement of your favorite work. Bœnninghausen's *Therapeutic Pocket Book,* a copy of which is in the library of nearly every homœopath, may be used by this plan, although it will be difficult from the fact of its briefness and the fact that the modalities of the part and of the generals are mixed together, to work your case to one remedy; but, rather, will you have to turn to your materia medica to differentiate between the last three or more remedies of your analysis.

In using Allen's *Slip Repertory* care must be taken not to give too high a standing to the nosodes or your final results will be apt to point to Psorinum or Tuberculinum.

The repertory was never made or intended to take the place of the materia medica; I cannot lay too great stress on the fact that it must never replace our constant study and use of the pathogenesis of our remedies, it should be used as an index to lighten the task of memory in storing the vast symptomatology of our remedies.

After the repertory has led us to the remedy which we believe covers our symptom picture, the selection of this remedy should be confirmed by reading its pathogenesis as given in one of our complete materia medicas. This not only acts as proof of the results obtained in the solving of our problems, but also acts as a check on hurried careless work and at the same time continually increases our knowledge of materia medica.

The use of the repertory is one of the higher branches of our art and before it can be mastered the laws governing the homœopathic treatment and cure of diseases, as given to us in the *Organon* and the *Chronic Diseases,* must be learned. Philosophy is rather like trying to explain a complicated problem of geometry to one who cannot use arithmetic, to try to teach the use of the repertory to one who does not comprehend Homœopathic Philosophy.

It is for this reason that I have begun this volume with a brief review of the *Organon,* as it applies to the repertory work, in the hope that this review will stimulate the desire for further and continued study of this first and greatest text-book of Homœopathy. I firmly believe that if Homœopathy is to survive in this age of therapeutic nihilism, when so many bastard practices are being fostered as Homœopathic, its survival will come from a comprehensive study of the *Organon*. Constantine Hering said: "If our school ever gives up the strict inductive method of Hahnemann we are lost and deserve only to be mentioned as a caricature in the history of medicine."

Homœopathy is from the beginning to the end an art of individualization. We have to individualize remedies and patients. However convenient it may seem to be, and however greatly it appeals to us, to think of our remedies in connection with diseases in the treatment of which they may be frequently called for, it must always be kept in mind that to allow our conception of our remedies to be limited by nosological terms will hinder us from utilizing our remedies to the fullest extent. To get the greatest good from the materia medica we must recognize our remedies as powerful curative agents ready to serve us in any case no matter what the name of the disease may be or what the laboratory findings may designate.

The analysis of forty remedies which is included in this work is in no way meant to replace your materia medica, but rather to help you to so systematize these remedies in your memory that they may be in shape to be readily called forth when occasion demands and that it may stimulate a desire to so study materia medica that in each of your cases the one remedy may be found which will serve you well, furnishing an effectual check upon poly-pharmacy and alternation of remedies.

It is not alone what the author has to offer to a reader that tells, it is what the reader can get out of the author, and in the last resort every homœopath must be his own materia medica maker. I think that you will be amply repaid for the time given to a careful study of this analysis, not only for the usable knowledge of the remedies that you will have acquired, but also,—and, perhaps, of the greatest importance, —the help it will be to you in enlarging and compiling your own materia medica.

I wish to take this opportunity of thanking Dr. G. G. Starkey, of Chicago, for the great assistance given me in revising and editing the proof of this work.

GLEN I. BIDWELL, M. D.

809 South Ave.,
    Rochester, New York.

How to Use the Repertory

Part I.

There are three things which merit the most careful consideration of the homœopathic practitioner—the taking of the case, the selection of the remedy and the administration of the remedy. The relations of these three steps are so closely intermingled, the one with the other, and the results of the one so dependent upon the care and accuracy with which the preceding steps have been taken, that I have presumed to call them the "Homœopath's Trinity."

Taking the Case.

Let us consider a moment the first division—that of taking the case. If we hope to attain even the smallest degree of success in the curative action of our remedies we must observe this first step closely and follow the instructions in the *Organon* (Secs. 83-104) carefully. If our case is indifferently taken or the wrong symptoms recorded we surely cannot proceed with the second step. No matter what process we take to arrive at the remedy, unless we have our case well taken we shall only have failure for our pains. Let us consider this most important step. What does it mean to take the case? I hear many answers to this: that everyone knows how to take the case, as it is simply a matter of recording the symptoms found in your patient. True, but what symptoms are you to look for and which are you to record? I will say with the utmost belief that less than one man in a hundred practicing Homœopathy to-day knows how to take a case properly. You may think that this is a pretty strong statement, but from my experience I think if any error has been made it is that I have placed the number too high. Many times I have had cases sent to me for repertory analysis with page after page of symptoms found in this patient, and out of this vast collection not one upon which a prescription could be hung, not one to differentiate this case from hundreds of others suffering from the same disease. There is the rub. There is the stumbling block. They all make a diagnosis and many of the cases sent to me would make fine text-book descriptions of the disease, but it is not the disease we want to make a record of; it is the individualized diseased patient. No man can make a homœopathic prescription from diagnostic or pathognomonic symptoms. The whole aim of the physician is to secure the language of nature. It is necessary to know sickness not from pathology, not from physical diagnosis, no matter how important these branches are, but by symptoms the language of nature.

In studying homœopathic philosophy as given in the *Organon*, the *Chronic Diseases* and Kent's *Lectures* we are struck by the fact that many of the main points are emphasized by arrangement of the ideas in groups of three, and it may not be out of place to review them briefly.

Three Injunctions.

Looking at the first two sections of the *Organon* we find the three injunctions—to cure promptly, mildly and permanently. Thus Hahnemann states the highest ideal of a cure which is the rapid, gentle and permanent restoration of health or removal of disease in its whole extent in the shortest, most reliable and harmless way. Let us consider what we mean by a cure. The physician who has not been trained in homœopathic philosophy answers that a cure consists of the disappearance of the pathological state. Does it? We believe not. For instance, does the removal of hæmorrhoids constitute a cure of the patient? If so, why do so large a percentage of operated cases return? Does the

2

removal of the carcinomatous breast cure the patient? If so, why do they return so frequently?
Does the removal of eruptions on the skin constitute a cure? If so, why are they followed by
various internal disorders which local measures
fail to relieve? No these are not cures. They
are simply the removal of the visible symptom
and one symptom does not make a picture of the
diseased patient. We must go back of this manifest symptom to the totality of this patient's
symptoms and take these into consideration when
making our prescription, and restore to health
by removing these symptoms; then the external
manifestations will disappear. There should always be an inward improvement when an external symptom has been made to disappear. If
the removal of symptoms is not followed by
restoration to health it cannot be called a cure.
In Sec. 70 we find the following: "All that a
physician may regard as curable in diseases consists entirely in the complaints of the patient and
the morbid changes of his health perceptible to
the senses; that is to say, it consists entirely in
the totality of symptoms through which the disease expresses its demand for the appropriate
remedy; while, on the other hand, every fictitious
or obscure internal cause and condition, or im-

aginary material, morbific matter are not objects of treatment."

Three Directions of Cure.

Another question that arises is: How can we demonstrate that we have cured and how may we know that our remedy is acting curatively? This leads us to consider the *three directions of cure*. We find that in order to produce a permanent cure symptoms must disappear from above downward—from within outward, and in the reverse order of their coming. All homœopaths who understand the art know that in order for the cure to be permanent the symptoms must go away in these directions. It is these directions that we must keep in mind when we treat an eruption on the skin, and see that the symptoms do not leave the skin and go to the brain, for if such a course is taken we know a mistake has been made, and if something is not done to make the symptoms take a proper course and go from the brain (center) to the skin (circumference) we are going to have a death certificate to fill out. Then when we treat a case of endocarditis, and after the administration of the remedy we observe a rheumatic swelling of the knee or ankle, and the patient will tell you, "This is the same sickness I had when Dr. So-and-So treated me for rheumatism before this heart trouble came on," you can be sure when this happens that you will make a cure, for the direction the symptoms have taken is according to the law, the symptoms have left the internals and have gone to the external parts, and if we leave the prescription alone a cure will result.

In Section 3 we have Hahnemann's statement of the THREE PRECAUTIONS, or those which I have called the "Trinity." He must perceive what is curable in disease; what is curative in medicine; and the application of the last to the first. And I can do no better than to quote Section three of the *Organon:* "The physician should distinctly understand the following conditions: What is curable in diseases in general, and in each individual case in particular; that is, the recognition of disease (*indicato*). He should clearly comprehend what is curative in drugs in general, and in each drug in particular; that is, he should possess a perfect knowledge of medicinal powers. He should be governed by distinct reasons in order to insure recovery by adapting what is curative in medicines to what he has recognized as undoubtedly morbid in a patient; that is to say, he should adapt it so that a case is

met by a remedy well matched with regard to
its kind of action (selection of the remedy, *in-
dicatum*), its necessary preparation and quantity,
and the proper time of its repetition. Finally,
when the physician knows in each case the ob-
stacles in the way of recovery, and how to remove them, he is prepared to act thoroughly,
and to the purpose, as a true master of the art of
healing."

Here Dr. Dudgeon's translation uses the word
"perceive," which means understand. We may
see a thing and not comprehend it; if we
perceive a thing we must understand it. Here
it is that our pathology and diagnosis will help
us. We know when we perceive structural
changes in tissues which have resulted in organic
destruction that the remedy will not replace tissue so destroyed. In these cases the only thing
we can do is to palliate the symptoms; but how
much more gently and surely we can do this with
our remedy than can be done by opiates, etc. If
there is any one thing that should convert a
family to Homœopathy it is to see the agonies
of a relative or friend relieved so they will still
retain their mental faculties until the last. Who
of us that have observed *Arsenicum* remove the
fear of death and the mental agonies of the last

hours that has not raised a silent prayer to our Maker for intrusting us with such a blessing for suffering humanity.

We must understand what is curative in medicine. How are we to do this? In Section 21 we find: "It is possible only to recognize the power of drugs to produce distinct changes in the state of feeling of the human body, particularly the healthy human body, and to excite numerous definite morbid symptoms in and about the same, and it follows that if drugs act as curative remedies they exercise this curative power only by virtue of their faculty of altering bodily feelings through the production of peculiar symptoms. Consequently those morbid disturbances, called forth by drugs in the healthy body, must be accepted as the only possible revelation of their inherent curative power." In this age of isopathy and serum therapy many are being led away by these will-o-the-wisps of allopathic teaching. One day we see a new serum or new bacterin or new vaccine; the next day some one comes along with something to remove the dangerous effects produced by their administration. These will go the way of all previous specifics and cure-alls advanced by the old school on experimental laboratory findings. Why is it their remedies come and go with almost the rapidity of a June frost? Simply because they are not based on a law. Where can we find anything in medicine that has had the lasting powers of the remedies proven by Hahnemann more than a century ago? They are still being used for the same symptoms and with the same success as when first given the profession. Let the old school perceive what is curative in their medicine according to the methods of Hahnemann instead of laboratory experiments, and they will have something lasting and of value.

The application of the remedy to the symptoms will be taken up fully under the repertory analysis of the individualized symptom picture, later in the paper.

The Three Miasms.*

The three chronic miasms are the next of the ideas we will consider. In sections 78-80 we find mentioned the three chronic miasms of Hahnemann. They are Psora, Syphilis and Sycosis. Here it is stated that if any of these three miasms is left to itself it will only become extinct with life itself. Surely with this statement no sane physician would deny the chronicity of any of

---

*Study the theoretiral part of Hahnemann's *Chronic Diseases.*

these miasms. It is in his *Chronic Diseases* that
Hahnemann tells us more fully concerning these
miasms.   For eleven years he observed and
studied with the tenacity, concentration and
ability for which his German habits and great
mind so well fitted him, before he brought forth
the theories of the miasms.   While there has
been much written against and a great deal' of
ridicule cast upon his theory of the psoric miasm,
those who have followed his teachings closely
believe in them, and from the knowledge thus
gained have been able to secure results in chronic
work which cannot be matched by those who
do not believe and who cast ridicule.   Whether
the psoric miasm has been the result of suppressed itch or not, and be that as it may, do not
waste your time in trying to throw it into disre-
pute, but when you have a case that will not
react to the apparently indicated remedy, look
well through your case and see if you cannot
discern one of the miasms.   Ofttimes you will
find traces and then the administration of the indicated anti-psoric will cause a reaction which
will lead to a cure.

In the dynamic, spirit-like, vital force, we find
the THREE PARALLELS of Hahnemann. Here we
again find that far-reaching, clear sightedness

and concise expression of Hahnemann's logic. Where have we since the writing of the *Organon* found anything which expresses that condition or being which controls and holds in harmony our life forces. Many of our physiologists and embryologists have given us theories concerning this condition but does the phagocyte theory or the opsonic theory with their variations give us anything better than Hahnemann's description? In Section 11 we find: "This vital force alone animating the organism in the state of sickness and of health imparts the faculty of feeling, and controls the function of life." Section 12: "Diseases are produced only by the morbidly disturbed vital force."

When first trying to master Homœopathy, after a perverted viewpoint gained in an old school college, this vital force was one of the hardest things for me to comprehend. In discussions raised from my standpoint as a pathologist and bacteriologist I would always chase my opponents to this stone wall, vital force, when they would nimbly hop over and intrench themselves behind this barrier, and I could only hurl my arguments against this wall and never dislodge them. In the light of advanced findings of our bacteriological laboratories I am inclined to believe that some of us carry this a little too far. While all fair minded physicians will admit that the predisposing cause of all diseases is the derangement of the vital force, I do not think we can deny that it has been proven beyond doubt that in the exciting cause of some diseases, at least, there is a bacteriological factor, and while we must admit that the ground must be made fallow by this deranged vital force in order for these minute vegetable organisms to produce their morbific effect, we must not pass over the fact that with this predisposing cause present the pathogenic bacteria are the exciting cause of many diseases.

In Sections 9-22 we find the explanation of the three parallels of force. These are as follows: (a) Plane of vital dynamis of organism; (b) Plane of disease cause; (c) Plane of medicinal substance.

In Section 83 Hahnemann gives us the THREE REQUIREMENTS or three qualifications necessary before we can properly examine a case. These are unbiased judgment and sound sense, attentive observation and fidelity in noting down the image of the disease. In the following paragraphs he further brings out these points by telling us that we must see, hear and observe. We must enter upon the work of taking our case with unbiased judgment and sound sense. This is the hardest requirement for all of us to follow, and one calling for [most] rigid self-scrutiny. How often it happens as we are listening to the symptoms of a case the picture of a remedy comes to mind, and if we do not use sound sense we are biased in favor of this remedy, and we do not question further and bring out the whole picture of the diseased patient. Then, again, we may maintain unbiased judgment until the case has been fully taken and then lose our sound sense of reasoning by saying such and such a case was like this and a certain remedy cured, therefore, "I will give that remedy without further investigation." Then, again, in younger men comes the desire to produce results quickly. They want to make a reputation to give relief from the pain at once, and so they give something of an opiate to deaden the pain, or they give some application to relieve the itching, or to dry up an eruption, although their sound sense tells them that a cure can never be made in this manner. And so in many ways we need to resist temptation and use sound sense and judgment freed from bias.

LET THE PATIENT TALK.

The next most important requirement is attentive observation. If we hope to arrive at the truth we must not only be attentive to what the patient tells us, and to what the nurse or family may impart, but we must observe closely the appearance of the patient himself. Ofttimes the symptom which will lead us to the remedy will be one which we may get by observation. The way the patient lies, sits, walks, talks, conducts himself generally, the appearance of discharges, the color of the eyes, hair, tongue, skin, etc., all have their place and are of the greatest importance in our record. Upon your powers of observation will depend not only the first image of your case but also your success in conducting the case after the first prescription has been made.

Three Mistakes.

The last group of three relating to the taking of the case will be the three mistakes made in examining the case, interruption of patient, asking direct questions and making answers conform to some remedy we may have in mind. A thing of the greatest importance in securing an image of a sickness is to preserve in the simplest form what the patient tells you.

Let him tell it in his own language, and unless he disgresses too much from the subject do not interrupt, for by so doing you may lose a line of thought and not be able to get him back to it again. Then do not ask direct questions. You must never put answers into your patients' mouths. You need to know all these particulars but without asking about it directly. Nine times out of ten the answer to a direct question will be "yes" or "no;" such answers are without value and should not be included in the record. Questions which give a choice of answers are also defective. Making answers conform to some remedy we may have in mind: a patient comes in, tells us a few symptoms; we immediately think of a remedy and begin to ask questions, and see if we cannot get enough evidence to convict him of *Belladonna*, *Arsenicum* or whatever it may be. It is surprising how well we can make the patient give us the symptoms we are looking for, as well as how little evidence it takes for some of us to make the conviction and give the remedy. We are more apt to blunder along this line if we do not write out our cases. The mere writing of the symptoms helps us to keep cool and not pass hasty judgment. On page 206 Tafel's translation of Nature of Chronic Diseases we find "The physician can, indeed, make no worse mistake than to consider too small the dose which I (forced by experience) have reduced after manifold trials and which are indicated with every antipsoric remery. Secondly, the wrong choice of a remedy, and, Thirdly, the hastiness which does not allow each dose to act its full time."

In remarking as to the cause of the second mistake we will quote from the same writings, on page 207, as follows:

"As to the second chief error in the cure of chronic diseases (the unhomœopathic choice of medicine) the homœopathic beginner (many, I am sorry to say, remain such beginners their life long) sins chiefly through inexactness, lack of earnestness and through love of ease."

A difficulty may arise in those obscure cases the symptoms of which have been masked by drugging, homœopathic and otherwise, operations, etc., so that these cases only present a few common symptoms, which can only guide us to a group of remedies in which the similimum must be found after exhaustive study of the materia medica.

Many times in these cases before we can make any progress we must go back through the life of the patient to childhood and note all symptoms which preceded the pathological change that now obscures the image of your case. "Symptoms that existed in childhood and since childhood and those present before any pathology existed are the corresponding symptoms of causes; as all causes are continuous into effects. They give us an image of the case from causes to pathological endings. These symptoms through childhood down to present are greatly important and describe the progress of sickness."

How to Find the Remedy.

Having thus far outlined, in a brief way, the homœopathic philosophy of the first division of our Trinity, we will pass to the second angle, that of finding the homœopathically indicated remedy.

We believe that Homœopathy is applicable to every curable case; the great thing is to know how to find and apply it.

If we had nothing but the mass of symptoms as recorded in the materia medica to help in the search for the single remedy which would cover the totality of a complicated chronic case, it would indeed be a gigantic task, and the excuse of many practitioners that they do not have the time to practice straight Homœopathy would be plausible; but we have in the repertory a valuable

help along this line, so that with little practice
and study the remedy may be found with amaz-
ing rapidity.

That the technique of surgery is wonderful in
its results when carefully applied in its proper
sphere is admitted by all physicians; that there
is an equally wonderful technique of scientific
Homœopathy must also be conceded or the reason for our being, as homœopaths, ceases to exist.
That the science of Homœopathy is exact when
applied by the use of the repertory has been
proved many times, and it will be my object to-
day not only to demonstrate this truth, but to try
and give you an insight into the methods used, so
that you may obtain accurate scientific results
easily and rapidly.

There are several complete repertories now
published and the use of any one of them will
be of untold aid in finding the right remedy.
When one has become familiar with their arrangement all the time that is really consumed is
in the taking of the case.

When you have decided on the repertory you
wish to use confine yourself to that one and completely master its arrangement, for the most
rapid work and the best results can only be obtained by the close study and working knowledge

of one. Personally, I can do the best and most rapid work with Kent's great work, and my demonstration here will be taken from Kent's *Repertory*. Before trying to use the repertory in your work read the headings of the general rubrics from beginning to end and thus familiarize yourself with the arrangement of the work, so that no time will be lost in looking for your symptoms. Only by this and by constant use can the repertory be a companion and helper.

Index to Arrangement of Kent's Repertory.

The *Repertory* is divided into the following thirty-seven sections, and are found in the order given below:

3

Tongue (found in many particulars). Gums are also covered by many particulars.

Taste, 426; Speech, 423.

Teeth, 435.

Throat, 452.

External throat, 474 (covers Glands, Pain, etc.).

Stomach, 478.

General symptoms referred through Stomach found under:

Appetite, 478 (which covers Hunger).

Aversion, 482.

Desires, 485.

Thirst, 529.

Particulars, as Nausea, 506; Eructations, 491, and Vomiting, 532.

Abdomen, 542.

Rectum, 605.

Constipation, 605; Diarrhœa, 608.

Stool, 633.

Urinary organs, 643.

Bladder, 643; Urination, 653.

Kidneys, 660.

Prostate Gland, 665.

Urethra, 667.

Urine, 678.

Genitalia (Male), 691.

Genitalia (Female), 712.

Abortion, Desires, Itching, Leucorrhœa (719), Menopause, Menses (721), Metrorrhagia, Tumors are all grouped under this section in alphabetical order.

Larynx and Trachea, 742.

Croup, Irritations and Voice are found here.

Respiration, 756.

Cough, 771.

Expectoration, 803.

Chest, 813.

> Hæmorrhage, Murmurs, Heart, Mammæ, Character of Milk, Palpitation are found in this section.

Back, 872.

Extremities, 937.

Sleep, 1200.

> Dreams, Comatose, Waking and Yawning are found here.

Chill, 1224.

Fever, 1242. (Types are arranged alphabetically.)

Perspiration, 1257.

Skin, 1267.

Generalities, 1364.

The two most important sections are found first in the book (MIND) and the GENERALITIES which are last. The Alpha and Omega, the beginning and the end.

Many of our chronic cases may be worked out from these two sections, from the mentals and the generals, as when these are found to be covered by one remedy the particulars, which have been observed, and many of the common symptoms will be found to fit in perfectly.

The same arrangement of each section is used throughout the book so that the sequence once understood the finding of any rubric is very simple.

First.—Time.

Second.—Conditions, in alphabetical succession.

Third.—Where there is condition of PAIN it is arranged as to:—

(a) Locality.

(b) Character.

(c) Extension.

To illustrate, take a mental symptom Restlessness (page 72):

Restlessness in general, under which are found all those remedies which have developed restlessness in the provers or removed the symptom clinically.

Then as to time.—Day time; morning; forenoon; afternoon; evening; night; midnight, and at some special hour.

Then conditions under which restlessness has been observed (given in their alphabetical order).

Aggravation in open air; driving out of bed; during chill; after dinner; during heat; before, during and after menses; mental labor; during perspiration; on waking; while sitting, and many others.

All these "modalities," when markedly present in a case, have great selective value.

Let us now examine the section on Generalities. Here we find aggravations, ameliorations, sensations and reactions of the patient, as a whole, to some physical condition, and to pain in general.

Under these rubrics where nothing is specified, aggravation is understood. The arrangement of the generalities is the same as throughout the other sections.

First, time—morning; noon; night; at particular portion of, and at particular hour.

After time follow general conditions of patient as whole in alphabetical order. (Aggravations and ameliorations of various parts, head; eye; ear; nose; face; stomach; chest; back; extremities; skin, etc., each is found in the section referring to that part in particular.)

These general aggravations as found under this last section are as follows: Better and worse from ascending; bathing; from cold; from wet and dry; from position; from motion and rest; from pressure; from rubbing, etc.

Under aggravation from cold we have the following particulars: Cold in general; cold air; becoming cold; cold, dry weather; entering a cold place; tendency to take cold; cold, wet weather; cold feeling in blood vessels, bones and inner parts.

In looking for aggravations from wet and dry we find under wet: Applications; getting wet; feet; head; perspiration; weather.

Aggravations and ameliorations as to weather conditions and time of year under: Weather and Autumn, warm, wet weather (under Warm); Summer, Storms, as to approach of and during; Spring, wet weather under Wet; Wind as to cold, warm south, windy and stormy weather; cold, dry and cold, wet weather is found under Cold.

Under this section we find the general character of Pain as to its onset and its disappearance (gradual or sudden).

Its character, as burning; constricting; digging; drawing; jerking; pinching; pressing; stitching; tearing, etc.

Its direction as to across; downward; inward; outward; upward.

We find inserted alphabetically throughout generalities nearly all the pathological nomenclature that there is in the book. Here are listed such rubrics as Anæmia; Arsenical poisoning; Atrophy; Cancerous affection; Caries; Chlorosis; Chorea; Convulsions (various forms); Dropsy; Faintness (fainting); Glands; Measles; Mercury, abuse of; Obesity; Quinine, abuse of; Scarlet fever; Syphilis, etc.

The character and frequency of the Pulse are found in this section, and it is grouped alphabetically as abnormal; frequent; intermittent; small; slow; full; hard; soft; tense; weak, etc.

Perspiration as to general effect is found here as giving no relief; aggravation after, amelioration after, and suppression of.

The characteristics and particulars of perspiration are found under that Section, page 1257.

Aggravations from eating and drinking and from different foods and drinks, as bacon; beer; bread; butter; fruit; meat; milk; pastry; tea, etc., the kinds and condition of food and drink, as cold drinks; cold food; dry food; frozen food; hot; rich; salt; sweet; sour and warm drinks and foods. These are all found under foods, while the desires, cravings and aversions to various foods and drinks, hunger and thirst (these being expressed by sensations from the stomach) are found under desires and aversions in the stomach section, page 478.

The general aggravations and ameliorations before, during and after menses are found in the generalities, while all important particulars and common menstrual symptoms are found under Section GENITALIA, FEMALE, page 712.

Many particulars having menstrual modalities will be found scattered through all sections of the book, as, for instance, Headaches with menstrual modifications, will be found under Head section. Abdominal distress modified by menses, in Abdominal section. Backache modified by menses under pain in back section, and so on through all conditions.

Through everything throughout the book the same arrangement exists. The aggravation or amelioration of patient as a whole is found under generalities, but when referred to a part or an organ its aggravation or amelioration is always found in its place under the section dealing with that particular part.

Pain.—One of the most frequent symptoms

that the physician is requested to remove is pain, and where to find the particular pain symptom in the repertory is most bewildering, unless we are familiar with its arrangement. The plan here is the same as elsewhere, which always carries one from what is more general to what is most particular in its minutest detail. The first list of remedies will be found to cover the time of occurrence. Second, all conditions under which the pain is observed, these are arranged in alphabetical order so that any particular condition may be readily found. Third, the locality of the pain. Fourth, the character of the pain, and last, the part or direction to which the pain extends. Keep this arrangement in mind and you will have no trouble finding that for which you search.

To illustrate, let us examine pain in the extremities, which is the longest and most complicated of all the pain sections.

First (page 1022) we have a list of remedies which have been found to have symptoms of pain in extremities.

Following this are two short rubrics, Right then Left, and Left then Right. Then follows condition as to time, and then a long list of conditions arranged alphabetically, under which pain

in extremities is found, as, before and during
chill; after slight exertion; during menses; on
motion; rheumatic; syphilitic; wandering, etc.

Then follows a list which localizes in general,
as Pain in Bones, in flexor Muscles; Joints; Nails;
Upper limbs; Shoulder; Upper arm; Elbow;
Forearm; Wrist; Hand; Fingers, and Thumb.
These subdivisions of upper arm are all worked
out under same general arrangement, as to time,
condition and extension to different parts. Cold;
heat; damp; dry; position and motion, as they
aggravate and ameliorate in particular, are all
found in their alphabetical order.

Then follow the lower limbs, which are divided
into their respective parts and which are treated
as to time, condition, etc., exactly as the upper
limbs. Thus having covered localities in general we proceed to deal with the character of the
pain in its various divisions.

Here, again, the whole extremities are
analyzed, as under Pain Burning (page 1067);
Burning generally, with its time and other conditions.

Burning in the joints and nails.

Burning in upper limbs generally, with time,
conditions and extremities.

Burning in all the localities of upper limbs, in

each instance with the time, modalities, conditions and extension. Then follow the burnings in the localities of the lower extremities arranged in the same way.

After one characteristic has been gone through exhaustively it passes on to the next kind of pain each in alphabetically order.

Pain whether in head, stomach, abdomen, chest or other part of body is gone through in this same general way into all its exhaustive finalities. This arrangement is so important that it will bear repetition.

First, Pain Generally: As regards time and conditions, ALWAYS IN ALPHABETICAL ORDER.

Second. Pain localized with regard to time, condition and extension.

Third. Character of pain generally with regard to time, conditions and extension.

Fourth. Character of pain as related to each locality in its turn (alphabetically) with continued reference to time, conditions and extension.

It is well to remember one point in looking for symptoms in the repertory, and that is, when you cannot find the symptoms as given in the language of the patient, do not despair and throw down the book in disgust, but look for some synonym until you find what you are looking for, and when you have found this make a cross reference in your repertory so it will be easier the next tmie.

Again, many fail to use the repertory because they think of symptoms in pathological terms. Symptoms are recorded in the materia medica in the language of the provers who were mostly laymen, and as the repertory is simply an index to the materia medica the rubrics must be in their simple language.

From Generals to Particulars.

Why do we work from generals to particulars? If a case is worked out merely from particulars it is more than probable that the remedy will not be seen and frequent failure will result. This is due to the fact that the particular directions in which the remedies in the general rubric tend have not been observed, and thus to depend upon a small group of remedies relating to some particular symptom is to shut out the other remedies, which may have that symptom, although not yet observed. By working the other way, from the generals to the particulars, the general rubric will include all the remedies that are related to the symptom.

Before the physician can make any suitable

homœopathic prescription we must take our case properly; this is true if we use a repertory or not, but is of the greatest importance if the repertory is to be used. Hahnemann gives clear and concise instructions for the taking of the case in the *Organon,* sections 83-104. Write out all the mental symptoms and all the symptoms and conditions pertaining to the patient himself, and search the repertory for the symptoms that correspond to these. Then individualize the case still farther by using the particular symptoms relating to the organs, sensations and functions, always giving an important place to the time of occurrence of every symptom. In this way we will have before us an individualized symptom-picture, not of the disease we wish to treat, but of the diseased patient we desire to cure.

Individualization of the symptom-picture and knowing which symptoms to give the most attention form the hardest part of the prescriber's armamentarium to acquire; and this process of logic, reasoning or whatever you may call it can only be obtained by study and application. The homœopathic physician must use discrimination, must individualize things dissimilar in one thing and yet similar in other ways. This is done by the generals, for without the generals of a case

no man can practice Homœopathy; without these
he will not be able to individualize and see dis-
tinctions. After gathering all the particulars of
the case one strong general rules out one remedy and rules in another. If you know your
materia medica you will at once see how to get
the generals and this will enable you to distinguish the remedy best adapted to the constitution
when two or more remedies have one symptom
in an equal degree. Then, again, a patient may
bring out particular symptoms so strange that
they have never been observed in the remedy;
but if the drug covers the generals it will not
only relieve those special symptoms, but cure
your case.

Remember this great truth, that the totality of
the symptoms as represented in the symptom-
picture of the prescriber will be an entirely different picture from that made by the surgeon, diag-
nostician or pathologist. No man who can only
understand the morbid anatomy and pathognomonic symptom can make a homœopathic prescription. It is from this difference as to inter-
pretation of the symptoms by the different special-
ists that the reporting of cases cured by the prescriber causes so much dissatisfaction. They
want to know the exact pathological condition

of each organ that produced the symptoms which were removed by the remedy; but the disease itself is only of benefit to the prescriber in helping him to select his grades of symptoms.

After we have our individualized symptom-picture before us we are ready to prepare the picture for repertory analysis. In order to analyze our case with rapidity we must go about it logically; we must have a starting place and a place to end. The start is made with the generals, and the particulars end it.

About the value of symptoms. Looking to Kent we find that he uses three classes—generals, particulars and common, and in his repertory he divides each into three grades—first, second and third. The generals and particulars, you must remember, have the greatest importance in our prescription.

Let us stop a moment and see what explanation he gives of these classifications. Looking to his *Lectures on Homœopathic Philosophy* we find that as generals he includes all things that are predicated of the patient himself. Things that modify all parts of the organism are those that relate to the general state; the more they relate to internals that involve the whole man the more they become general. Many common symptoms may run into generals and particulars. Things that relate to the ego are always general. The patient says, Doctor, I am so thirsty; I burn so; I am so cold, etc.; the things he says he feels are always general. His desires and aversions are general; menstruation is general, for when a woman says I feel so and so during menses she has no reference to her uterus or ovaries; her state, as a whole, is different when she is menstruating. (*Homœopathic Philosophy,* p. 242.)

The general symptoms as such are often not expressed by the patient or are not always to be recognized at first to be so; but on examining a group or series of particular organs we find a certain modality or feature which runs so strongly through them that it may express the patient himself. Here we have a general composed of a series of particulars. This most often happens under character of pains, as cramping, burning, etc., or in conditions associated with pains as heaviness, numbness, etc. Here a symptom may be raised from a particular or even a common to a common general.

Generals Divided into Three Grades.

(A) Mentals; (B) Physical; (C) Things affecting the whole physical body. The first general group of symptoms which are of the highest value are the symptoms of the mind. These are divided into three grades: The Will; Perversions of understanding; Perversions of memory.

(A) The group of symptoms referred to the will are of first importance in individualizing your case for repertory study and are manifest through perversions of loves with various fears.

In sickness the patient's nature often becomes changed; the mental symptoms are manifest. They may be quarrelsome, angry, irritable, tearful, they may hate their loved ones, they may be fearful, intolerant of sympathy. These are often the most difficult of all symptoms to obtain as they are most often concealed from the world, from friends and their physician. Among symptoms of this group you will find ailments from anger, bad news, grief, love, joy, reproach, sexual excesses, contrariness, cursing, cowardice, hatred, irritability, jealousness, loquacity, quarrelsomeness, indifference, sadness, etc.

(B) Perversions of understandings as manifest in delusions, hallucinations and illusions, etc. These take the second place in value for repertory work. Among symptoms of this group, which are not self-explanatory of the above, are found: absorbed, clairvoyance, con-

4

fusion, dullness, comprehension, both difficult and easy; ecstacy, excitement, imbecility, mental activity, ailments from mental exertion, etc.

(C) Those of the lowest value of the mental symptoms are the perversions of memory. Such symptoms as absent minded, errors in answers, mistakes in writing and speech, disorders of speech, etc., are found in this group.

NOTE.—IF MENTAL SYMPTOMS ARE MARKED, ESPECIALLY IF IT IS A CHANGE FROM NORMAL, THEY ARE OF THE UTMOST IMPORTANCE TO THE CASE. GET THESE SYMPTOMS CLEAR, THE GIVE THEM THE HIGHEST STANDING IN YOUR REPERTORY ANALYSIS. THE REMEDY WHICH INCLUDES THEM WILL BE CURATIVE.

GROUP TWO—PHYSICAL.—The next symptoms of importance among the generals are grouped as those which apply to the physical generals that deal with physical loves and sensations of the body as a whole. These may be sub-divided into two groups:

(a) The highest rank should be given to perversions of the sexual sphere, including menstrual generals. Symptoms found under this group would be those with aggravations before, during and after menses; effect of coition, urination, etc.; character of discharges. (Taking the normal as our guide any change, a decrease or increase or perversion would constitute a symptom.)

(b) The next of importance would be those symptoms pertaining to appetite, food desires and aversions and thirst. (Eating and drinking as they affect the stomach are particular, but as they affect the body as a whole are general (as the craving for salt as found under *Natrum mur.*).

GROUP THREE.—Things affecting the entire physical body. Weather and climatic influences, foods that aggravate, extremes of temperature, positions, motions, etc., as they affect the body as a whole (as worse from standing under *Sulphur* and *Valerian* is a marked general of those remedies), are all generals as found in this group.

The effect of weather, climate and extremes of temperature are of great value, but are ofttimes difficult to get clearly. We must use great care in bringing out these symptoms if we are to rule out remedies thereby.

Many times we find patients stating, "I cannot stand heat," but on enquiry we find that they hate cold, but that their aversion is to warm, close and stuffy rooms, or it may be that they are worse in summer.

In many conditions, such as rheumatism, we would expect aggravation from weather changes, the absense of these modalities, or that they might be better in wet damp weather, would transfer this system from a general to a peculiar, particular or characteristic.

Such symptoms as refer to aggravation and amelioration from bathing, wetting, pressure, touch, rubbing, jarring, defecation, sleep, dreams, parts of day, time, month and seasons, are all generals.

Sides of the body as left and right, semi-lateral, oblique (appearance of symptoms as found in *Agaricus* and *Asclepias*), alternate sides, changing about from side to side or various parts of body, congestions, contractions, discoloration of parts, atrophy, chlorosis, etc., are all classed in this group of Generals.

Special senses are often so closely related to the whole man that a great many of their symptoms are general, as various odors make sick, the smell of cooking nauseates, the sight or smell of food sickens, oversensitiveness to sounds, noise, light, etc., would all be classed in this group.

Particular and Common Symptoms.

The generals always rule out non-agreeing particulars. Under the particular symptoms we find:

"The symptoms that are predicated of a given organ are things in particular. The symptoms that cannot be explained are often very peculiar. The more they relate to the anatomy of a part the more external they are; the more they relate to tissues the more liable they are to be particular, although many symptoms of regions are both common and particular. Symptoms are on a more or less sliding scale. What is peculiar in one remedy may be in no degree peculiar in another; for instance, it would not be peculiar to have a fever patient thirsty. It is a common thing for them to want to drink, but it would be peculiar to have a patient without fever or chilly who wanted to drink all the time, as we find in some chronic cases." (*Lectures on Homœopathic Philosophy*, pp. 237, 240.)

Under common symptoms we find: "All those which are common to both the drug and disease. That which is pathognomonic is always common. For instance, if we had a pleurisy it would be a common thing to want to keep the chest wall quiet and you would get the symptom worse from motion, one of the keynotes of *Bryonia;* but if there were no other symptoms of *Bryonia* present we could not make a prescription on that rubric alone. Again, if we had an abscess it would be a common thing for it to be sensitive, and if pus was forming we would have throbbing pains and redness, but *Belladonna* could not be given on these common symptoms if there were no other *Belladonna* symptoms present. You can readily see how the common symptoms have no place in our repertory work. You need not bother with the common symptoms, for when you have worked your case out from the generals and particulars turn to your materia medica and you will find the remedy will contain most of the common symptoms." (*Ibid.*, p. 238, 245.)

Grades of Particular and Common Symptoms.

After considering the generals we take up the symptoms referring to various parts or organs of the body. These are known as particulars, and are of lower value in repertory analysis than the generals.

Running through all symptoms from innermost to outermost, from mind to skin, from generals to particulars, we have two divisions:

(a) The strange, rare, peculiar and uncommon symptoms.

(b) The common symptoms.

Be these general or particular, mental or physical, common symptoms must be considered last in every case of repertory study. First, we must become familiar with symptoms that are common, then it will be easy to know what are uncomomn, strange, rare and peculiar.

Common symptoms as related to many remedies are found in the large rubrics in the repertory, such as constipation, irritability, chill, fever, sweat, weakness, etc. These common symptoms may become peculiar where their circumstances are peculiar, as trembling during stool, before a storm, during urination, etc. Chilliness, if constant, is a strong, common general, as it refers to the whole patient, but if it comes only in bed, or before urination or before, during or after stool or in relation to menses or only at night or while eating, it is at once changed to a strange, rare, peculiar or characteristic.

Weakness is also common if constant, but may become uncommon, strange, rare and peculiar if it comes only while eating, or during a storm or after stool or when cold.

All of these modalities are common to no known disease, and so they become striking and peculiar and help to individualize the picture for repertory work.

It is in showing what is common to disease that pathology helps us, hence it is important that we make a diagnosis, not that we may prescribe for the disease, *per se*, but to know what symptoms are common, and, therefore, worthless as individualizers.

The common diagnostic symptoms of typhoid fever are the general malaise, epistaxis, the peculiar temperature wave, gurgling and tenderness in the right iliac fossa, rose spots, early dicrotic pulse, enlarged spleen, Widal reaction of the blood, Diazzo reaction of the urine. These symptoms you use to make your diagnosis; you expect to find them in every case, but among them are no symptoms to lead you to a remedy.

Pathology through diagnosis helps us to eliminate many symptoms as result of disease. Stiffness may be a very troublesome symptom to your patient, but if it is the result of an ankylosed joint you know that remedies would not cure, therefore that symptom would be ruled out.

Pains due to pressure of tumors or growths in the abdomen are very troublesome to the patient, but we know that when such end products of disease exist, it is beyond the realm of medicine to cure without the removal of the offending growth. Thus all symptoms produced by pressure of the growth must be ruled out of the symptoms picture to be used in repertory analysis.

Kent says: "We must not expect a remedy

that has the generals must have all the little symptoms. It is a waste of time to run out all the little symptoms if the remedy has the generals. Learn to omit the useless particulars, the common particulars—common particulars are generally worthless. Get the strong, strange, peculiar symptoms and then see to it that there are no generals in the case that oppose or contradict."

Keynotes.

It is among the peculiar symptoms that we find the so-called keynotes that are used by so many prescribers who take three, (or many are content with but one) characteristic outstanding symptoms, ignoring all others and overlooking the fact that there must be a general relation between the symptoms of the patient and those of the remedy.

This keynote system of prescribing is highly attractive to many minds, because it looks so easy and does away with all tedious comparison of drugs and also from the fact that many brilliant cures were made by means of the keynotes in the hands of Lippe, Allen and other advocates of the system. But you must remember that these men, as well as any others who have been successful with keynotes, have had a keen enough perception into totalities and the patho-

genesis of remedies so that they used the keynote which was not ruled out by contradicting
general symptoms of the patient.

Many of the so-called keynotes are both general and particular (aggravation from motion
of *Bryonia* and sore, bruised sensations of
Arnica).

The great trouble with the keynotes is that
they are so often misused. Keynotes are often
valuable characteristic symptoms, but if these
keynotes are taken as final and the generals do
not confirm then failures will come.

Grades of Drug Symptoms.

The grades of the drug symptoms are desig-
nated in the repertory by the use of different
sized type. Kent uses three grades, Bœnninghausen had four, but this fourth grade is included in those of the third under Kent's classi-
fication. Distinction in the drug symptoms
by placing one in the first grade by using capi-
tals and heavy faced type; under the second
grade by using italics and under the third grade
by using small letters. Under the first grade
are included all those symptoms which were
brought out in every prover and that have since
been verified. Under the second grade those
symptoms which were brought out in the ma-

jority of provers and have since been verified, and under the third grade those symptoms which only a few of the provers developed, those symptoms which are clinical and which have since been verified.

Repertory Analysis, Dosage and Repetition.

After the longest and most difficult part of your task, that of individualizing your symptoms, has been completed the remaining portion, that of selecting your remedy with the repertory, is quickly done and is a simple mathematical proposition. Like all other mathematical problems we must start with the right premises and follow certain axioms in order to arrive at the correct solution. Thus if the logic of our symptom analysis be correct, if the technique of selection be without a flaw, the choice of the remedy must be mathematically certain.

Before giving the demonstration of the repertory analysis I wish to say a few words concerning the administration of the remedy after we have found the one which covers our individualized symptom picture. One of the most difficult things to comprehend is when to repeat the dose. You will find as a general thing in acute cases that if a slight aggravation of the symptoms comes in a short time you will not think of giving another dose, for your patient will get along better without more medicine; but there are conditions when it is necessary to repeat the dose. For this there is no clear-cut rule that can be laid down, and it is a very difficult thing to teach and to understand; rather it can only come by experience and by using your powers of observation. The safe rule to follow is, never repeat the dose after reaction begins. If more than one dose is necessary repeat the dose until there is an improvement and then stop; more doses would only retard the cure. When reaction is taking place never repeat the remedy; when reaction ceases or improvement stops the remedy may be repeated. Many good homœopathic prescriptions are spoiled by too oft repeated doses of the right remedy. We are often treating the effects of too many doses of the remedy when we think we are treating the disease. I do not like to bring the question of potency up in this place, but there is one thing I wish to emphasize; that is, when the dilution of the right remedy will only carry your case part way to health, and you are sure you have the right remedy, increase the strength of the remedy rather than change to another unsuitable one. In this way you will find your cases being carried on to a complete cure.

We find certain rules given us for the repetition of the remedy in our chronic diseases and Hahnemann discusses these on pages 209 to 213, in speaking of the third mistake in the treatment of the diseases. Quoting in part, we find, on page 209: "The third leading mistake that the Homœopathic physician cannot too carefully or steadfastly avoid is in hastily and thoughtlessly giving some other medicine . . . but if once a medicine . . . is acting well and usefully, which is seen by the eighth or tenth day, then an hour or even half a day may come when a modern homœopathic aggravation again takes place. The good results may not appear in their best light before the twenty-fourth or thirtieth day. The dose will probably have then exhausted its favorable action about the fortieth or fiftieth day, and before that time it would be injudicious and an obstruction to the progress of the cure to give any other medicine. Experience teaches that a cure cannot be accomplished more quickly and surely than by allowing the suitable antipsoric to continue its action so long as the improvement continues. . . . Whoever can restrain his impatience as to this point will reach his object the more surely and the more certainly . . . periods of aggravation will occur, but so long as only the original ailments are renewed and no new, severe symptoms present themselves, they show a continuing improvement, being homœopathic aggravations which do not hinder but advance the cure. The physician must; therefore, in chronic diseases, allow all antipsoric remedies to act thirty, forty or even fifty and more days by themselves, so long as they continue to improve the diseased state perceptibly to the acute observer, even though gradually; for so long the good effects continue with the indicated doses and these must not be disturbed and checked by any new remedy." In footnote, page 212, we find: "But he who will not allow himself to be convinced of this and imitate what I now teach, he who is not willing to imitate it exactly, can leave the most important chronic diseases uncured."

This third step of our Trinity is of equal importance with the first two, for no matter how well you have done the first and second parts of your task all your efforts can be spoiled by the wrong administration of the remedy.

When we have given our remedy on the above formula we may expect certain things to happen. In all curable cases we will expect a cure to take place or at least to be started. We may know that this cure is taking place by certain signs of nature which are given to us in the symptoms of the patient, and the way these signs or symptoms disappear will tell us if we are going to make a cure. If we are to cure the symptoms must disappear from above downward, from within outward and in the reverse order in which they came.

From the study of the *Organon* and the *Chronic Diseases*, we learn that there are certain other things that we may expect after the prescription has been made. Kent gives these observations as eleven in number. I will simply give them without further comment, as an explanation may be found in Kent's *Lectures on Homœopathic Philosophy*, or in a paper on the subject by myself, published in a late number of the *North American Journal of Homœopathy*.

Following the dose one of the following results is to be expected:

"1st. A rapid cure will take place with no aggravation of symptoms.

2d. The aggravation will be rapid, short and strong, and is followed by rapid improvement of the patient.

3d. A long aggravation with final and slow improvement of patient.

4th. A long aggravation with final decline of patient.

5th. Full time amelioration of symptoms with no special relief of patient.

6th. Amelioration comes first and aggravation comes afterward.

7th. Too short relief of symptoms.

8th. Old symptoms are seen to appear.

9th. New symptoms appearing after the remedy is given.

10th. Patients who prove every remedy given.

11th. That symptoms take the wrong direction."

The first case used will be an illustration of repertory analysis, working through the two divisions of Mental and Physical Generals. (Many are partial to this method, and it is well to use it in the beginning, as it trains you in the repertory arrangement.)

My examples, as further cases illustrated will show, does not follow this method and has laid me open to criticism (from some sources) of being too mathematical in my methods and of the liability of securing erroneous results. This criticism might be sustained if one depended upon the repertory as the final deciding factor for the remedy; but taking the pathogenesis of the remedy, as given in a complete materia medica, as the court of last resort I am at a loss to see where the criticism is justifiable. To me, at least, my method of taking the most prominent general, be it mental or physical, as a starting point and eliminating remedies from the group thus reached is much more comprehendable and more easily followed. In advocating this method I assume the physician to be familiar with the arrangement of his repertory and a master of the art of the individualization of cases.

Cases Illustrating Repertory Work

Mrs. C. F., 35 years, record contains the following symptoms:

MIND.—Thinks of nothing but death.

Homesick and worries about home whenever away.

Cross and irritable.

Memory very poor. Forgetful, which is very troublesome.

Company makes her nervous; does not want to stay and visit with friends when they come to call or spend the evening.

Imagines there are persons in the room.

Difficult to concentrate her thoughts on any one thing long enough to complete it.

HEAD.—Headache most of the time, severe pressure at base of skull.

5

Pain in right side of head extending down to neck.

Aggravation from warmth of bed; from mental exertion.

Amelioration from lying.

Itching of scalp with much dandruff, with falling of hair.

Vertigo in hot room and when rising from seat.

STOMACH.—Hungry all the time, but a little satisfies.

Much belching of tasteless gas.

Desires sweets which disagree.

ABDOMEN.—Sensitive to pressure of clothing.

Much rumbling of flatus with pressure both up and down.

URINATION.—Profuse, pale and alkaline.

Sometimes burning in bladder after urination.

MENSES.—Profuse.

Irregular.

Dark, with dark clots.

Very much depressed and inclined to be tearful before menses.

Leucorrhœa profuse for few days after menses —excoriates.

SLEEP.—Good but unrefreshing. Wakens tired and exhausted.

Very sleepy after dinner (at night).

Dreams frightful, usually of drowning.

GENERAL AGGRAVATIONS AND AMELIORATION.
—Better in open air.

Worse from pressure of clothes about abdomen and throat.

Very sensitive to noise.

Repertory Analysis.

MENTALS.—IMAGINES PHANTOMS, ETC. (page 27.)—*Ambr., Apis, Arg. m., Ars.,* BELL., *Carbo v., Caust., Crot. h., Hep., Hyos.,* LACH., *Lyc., Merc., Nat. m., Op., Phos., Samb., Stram., Thuj., Sulph., Zinc.*

SENSITIVE TO NOISE (page 79).—*Apis, Ars.,* BELL., *Carbo v., Caust., Lach., Lyc., Merc., Nat. m., Op., Phos., Zinc.*

AVERSION TO COMPANY (page 12).—*Bell., Lach., Lyc., Nat. m.*

PHYSICAL GENERALS—AMELIORATION FROM OPEN AIR (page 1307).—*Lach., Lyc., Nat. m.*

MENSES DARK (page 723).—*Lach., Lyc.*

MENSES IRREGULAR (page 724).—*Lach., Lyc.*

MENSES DARK CLOTTED (page 722).—*Lycopodium.*

Therefore, if our analysis has been correct *Lycopodium* should cover this case in its entirety, and consulting our Materia Medica we find not only the general symptoms of the case that we have used in our analysis but all the others which are recorded in the record of the case. Therefore, we know that this remedy is the similimum to the case, and if administered carefully will cure.

The second case that I will give will show you how not to use the repertory. This method of trying to find a remedy which will cover every symptom of the patient is the one most of you try to use, and it is one that is discouraging not only from the fact that it takes so much time, but as well from the fact that many times the repertory will not give the particular rubric for which you may be looking. I selected this case for the reason that each of the symptoms can be found in the repertory and that one remedy covers them all.

CASE 2.—Mrs. H. S. came to me 2-12-'07 with the following symptoms which I will give in her own language: "I am so nervous; am afraid I shall kill some of my people, as I go all to pieces and can't control myself. Thinking about killing, I dream of killing my little girl. If I do not get better soon I shall commit murder. Every afternoon I have pain over my eyes as if burned. Can't read at night, as there are sharp pains going through my eyes; if I persist in reading dark points appear on the page so I cannot see the print. Hungry most of the time; in morning when I awaken there is burning pain in my stomach which grows worse until I get up, when it goes away. Always have to take pills to move my bowels; before they move there is a sharp cutting pain in the rectum and many times the bowels come out while at stool. If I drink beer will have piles for two or three days. My menses have been too often since my last child, three years ago, and for a week before I am sick have whites each morning, which are much worse walking. There is not much flow, and it only lasts two or three days and smells sour as vinegar. Can't sew for past month, as there are stitching pains in the back of my neck when bending my head forward. Feet cold as ice every afternoon and the cramps in my calves keep me awake nearly all night. Do not shop, as I feel so badly when I have to stand long."

REPERTORY ANALYSIS.—Fear of killing people. —*Abisn., Ars. a., Nux v., Rhus t., Sulph.*

Dreams of committing murder.—*Rhus t., Sulph.*

Burning pains over the eyes, worse afternoon. —*Sulph.*

Sharp shooting pains at night, on reading.—*Phyto., Sulph.*

Followed by dark points.—*Con., Sulph.*

Burning pains in stomach on waking, better rising.—*Sulph.*

Cutting pain in rectum before stool.—*Asar., Sep., Sulph.*

Prolapsus recti during stool.—*Ign., Lyc., Podo., Rhus t., Sulph.*

Leucorrhœa mornings, worse walking.—*Nat. m., Bov., Sarsa., Sep., Sulph.*

Menses scanty, short duration.—*Amm. c., Lach., Puls., Sulph.*

Menses smell sour.—*Carbo v., Sulph.*

Stitching pain in neck from bending head forward.—*Sulph.*

Feet cold afternoon.—*Nux v., Sulph.*

Cramps in calves while in bed.—*Ars. a., Caust., Ign., Sulph.*

Worse standing—*Con., Cycl., Lil. t., Puls., Sep., Sulph., Valer.*

Here we see that *Sulphur* covers each symptom, but with a good knowledge of the arrangement of the repertory it took me some time to work it out. Now to demonstrate how much more rapidly we can arrive at the same results by working from the generals to particulars, we will start with a general rubric:

Menses scanty, short duration.—We find the following nineteen remedies that have this symptom in the first and second grades: *Alum., Am-c., Asaf., Bar. c., Cocc., Dulc., Graph., Lach., Mang., Merc., Nat. m., Nux v., Phos., Plat., Puls., Sepia, Sulph., Thuj.*

Now among this group of nineteen remedies will be found one which will cover the totality of our case. If we were to give a remedy upon this one symptom alone we might give any of the above, for they all have this condition in a high degree; but if we did not give the right one we should not cure the case. We must individualize our case still further, so we will use another general.

Worse standing.—In consulting the repertory we find that of the first nineteen there are only the following seven which have the symptom in the first or second grade: *Con., Cocc., Phos., Plat., Puls., Sep., Sulph.*

But still we have seven remedies, any one of which may be the remedy so far, and we must individualize still further by another symptom. We will take the general, better in open air. Here we find that we have only four remedies of our previous group which have this symptom in the first and second grade—*Con., Phos., Puls., Sulph.*

We have now worked our list down to four remedies and we will individualize again by taking another general, fear of committing murder. This gives us *Sulphur*, the only remedy which covers all of the symptoms we have taken so far. Now if the logic of our reasoning be correct, if the technique of selection be without a flaw, *Sulphur* must be the mathematically correct remedy, and reference to the pathogenesis of the remedy shows that *Sulphur* not only covers these four symptoms we have used, but it also contains all the other particular and common symptoms of the case. The proof of the pudding is in the eating, so we will turn to our record and we find that patient was discharged 7-7-'07; that all symptoms had disappeared, bowels move naturally. Says she never felt better in her life.

CASE 3.—Boy, age 14; epileptic attacks for three years. First attack followed fright caused by other boys' make believe to hang him. Attacks increasing in frequency until at this time they occur every two weeks. The following symptoms were given: Attacks begin by running around in circle, then falls down unconscious. Attacks are more frequent in cold dry weather and during new moon. Involuntary urination during the attack. Boy complains of always being cold; wants to keep warm both summer and winter. He is very touchy; everything makes him cry; seems depressed all the time. Appetite either ravenous or wanting. Aversion to all kinds of sweets, of which he was previously very fond.

REPERTORY ANALYSIS.—Under complaint caused by fright we find thirty-six remedies. Of these the following twenty-one have the symptoms on the first and second grade: *Acon., Apis, Arg. n., Art. v., Aur., Bell., Caust., Coff., Cupr., Gels., Glon., Hyos., Ign., Lach., Lyc., Nat. m., Nux v., Op., Plat., Puls., Rhus t.*

Sadness and depressed.—*Acon., Arg. n., Aur., Bell., Caust., Gels., Ign., Lach., Nat. m., Plat., Puls.*

Worse cold dry weather.—*Acon., Caust.*

Aversion to sweets.—*Causticum.*

We have arrived at the solution of the case by four steps and have used all general symptoms. Now you may ask, why did we start with the rubric complaints caused by fright? First: This is a general symptom and we are working from the generals to particulars. Second: This condition was caused in this boy by fright. This mental shock was so profound that it caused the whole condition of this patient to be changed.

It not only produced the epileptic seizure, but affected his desires as well. Some one of the remedies found under this rubric will be the one which will cover the totality of the case. The second symptom we will take is another general—sadness and depression. We take this rubric from the fact that it is a mental condition produced by a derangement of the patient's most internal condition, the mind. Now if we hope to cure this case we must have a remedy which has produced this symptom in the provers, so among our first twenty-one we find eleven with this symptom in the first and second grade. Another general condition is the modality that the attacks are worse in cold dry weather. Among the eleven remedies found in the first two rubrics we find only two which are worse in cold dry weather. In order to decide which of these two will cover our case we will take the general aversion to sweets. Here we find that *Causticum* is the only remedy which covers our rubrics. If our reasoning has been correct, if the technique of selection is without a flaw, *Causticum* must be the mathematically correct remedy, and turning to our materia medica we find that the pathogenesis of *Causticum* not only contains the rubrics we have used in our analysis, but the remaining symptoms of our case as well. Therefore, *Causticum* is the remedy we will give. Our records show that two doses of this remedy were administered with the following results: The attacks lessened during the first month to one; the second attack, a very slight one, did not follow for seven weeks, and now, after an interval of a year and a half, there has been no sign of a return, so we may safely say the boy is cured.

CASE 4.—Mrs. A. S., æt. 28; married four years; menses have always been irregular, but during the first year of married life were more regular but always profuse. The third year married gave birth to a seven-pound child; labor normal; no lacerations. Since labor has never been well; the menses would appear every two weeks; then every five or six weeks, with no regularity. The flow would be profuse and weakening. Had had curettages and various treatments without any relief. The condition of patient at the time of first prescription was as follows: Menses irregular and profuse; great weakness when walking; the walk from the car to office completely exhausted her. Cannot sleep; what sleep she gets is unrefreshing. No appetite; does not want to think of eating.

Craves beer, of which she had never tasted but once, and then it was repulsive. Sweats easily; is in a perspiration most of the time and has to be very careful about getting in a draft, as when she becomes chilly she is nauseated.

REPERTORY ANALYSIS.—Menses irregular and profuse—*Apis, Arg. n., Art. v., Benz. ac., Calc. c., Carb. ac., Caust., Cimi., Cocc., Con., Dig., Ign., Iod., Ip., Iris., Kreos., Lyc., Murex, Nux v., Nux m., Secale, Sepia, Staph., Sulph., Tuberc.*

Worse from warmth.—*Arg. n., Calc, c., Cocc., Con., Ign., Iod., Ip., Lyc., Nux m., Sulph.*

Extreme weakness when walking.—*Calc. c., Cocc., Con., Iod., Lyc., Nux m., Sulph.*

Great desire for beer.—*Calc., Cocc., Sulph.*

Nauseated when chilly.—*Cocculus.*

Just a word in explanation of our selection of the rubrics in this case. Why did we start with the symptom, menses irregular and profuse? In the first place, it is a general symptom; then it is the symptom above all others that has proved the change in the patient's general condition; if we expect to cure this case we must have a remedy that has in its symptomatology this condition. On the other hand, if we took any of the remedies we find in the first and second grades under this rubric we would have a remedy for this local condition that so many and various lines of treatments had been used upon with no results; so not only must we take this symptom, but must take the other symptoms, which make this case of irregular and profuse menses different from every other case of the same condition; in other words, that makes of it an individual case. Therefore, we proceed with the other symptoms.

One word more, about our fourth rubric—great desire for beer. Ordinarily this symptom would be of little value, but here we find a patient that before she was affected with this change of internal conditions did not like beer; in fact, she had never tasted it but once and then it was repulsive to her, but now she is sick; some change in her desires has produced a condition of her economy whereby she has a craving for beer. Now the condition has changed and a symptom which in other cases would be of little or no value deserves a prominent place in our record analysis.

This case also has another interesting peculiarity, in that if the keynote prescribers had been working at it they might have reached a correct solution, for in this case we find that the particular symptom, nauseated when chilly, is found under only one remedy, *Cocculus*.

Our selection of *Cocculus* in this case was justified, for the case was cured. The menses became regular and normal; the weakness disappeared; the craving for beer vanished; the excessive perspiration and nausea left, until after four months she was discharged stating that she never felt so well in her life.

There are some cases where we cannot individualize closely enough to work our case down to less than two or three remedies. When this occurs we take that remedy which has the symptoms in the highest grade and if the pathogenesis of the drug justifies we give that. To illustrate, I will give the analysis of a case without the history.

Menses copious and dark.—*Am. c., Am. m., Ant. c., Ars. a.,* BELL., *Bism., Bov., Bry., Calc. c., Calc. p., Carbo a.,* CHAM., *China, Cimic., Cocc.,* CROC., *Cycl., Ferr., Graph., Ign., Kali n., Kreos., Lach., Lil. t., Mag. c., Nit. ac.,* NUX M., *Nux v., Phos., ac.,* PLAT., PULS., *Sabin., Sec., Sep., Sulph.*

Worse riding in a wagon.—COCC., *Ign., Nux m.,* SEPIA, *Sulph.*

Worse before menses.—*Nux m.,* SEPIA, SULPH.

. Aversion to milk.—*Sepia, Sulph.*

Sadness in evening.—SEPIA, *Sulph.*

Vertigo looking down.—*Sepia,* SULPH.

Here we find by giving a numerical value of two to those of the first grade and of one to the second grade that we have *Sepia* having a value of nine and *Sulphur* a value of eight.

Absolute reliance cannot be placed on numerical superiority of points for any one remedy; that is, a remedy not having so many points as another will yet have the better correspondence with the vital features of the symptom picture, and be the curative drug to select. This selection must be made from a final comparison of the drug's pathogenesis as given in a complete materia medica.

In closing the cases for analysis I wish to conclude with the following case to illustrate two points. 1st. That, as regards our prescription, diagnosis has little or nothing to do. 2d. That if we could all forget our diagnosis while taking our case for a prescription we should all be able to do better work. This case will be given as taken by a young lady who had never studied medicine; in fact, all she knew concerning that subject was that when she or her friends were sick she wanted a homœopathic remedy to make them well. I have never seen this case personally, but know she is well from reports that I have received through the mail.

Mrs. H. C., æt. 42; widow. Has eruption on legs, which burns and itches, and is worse from warmth of bed. She cannot keep her legs quiet at night. Is worse from warmth of stove, which causes creeping sensation over whole body. Feet are icy cold during day, but soles burn at night in bed. Lameness of left shoulder, which has lasted since rheumatism four years ago; this is worse when lying on it. The hands go to sleep and feel numb, more especially the left one. The wrist pains as if sprained when awakening. All pains are of burning character and change locality often and suddenly.

Sometimes there are small ulcers on inner side of left thigh, from which there is a thin offensive discharge; walking will cause them to smart, become red and puffy. Stiffness in small of back on bending or beginning to move. The pains go down the thigh. She has a dry cough, which is worse after sleep and is caused by a tickling in the throat. This cough has always come the last of March or the first of April, and would last until real hot weather had come; with this cough she is quite hoarse and has sensation of lump in the throat. Menstruation is dark and scanty and offensive; has not been regular since last child, twelve years ago; she says all her aches and pains are better during her flow, and she never feels so well as when flowing freely, although it is sometimes accompanied by a painful diarrhœa. At other times she is always constipated; has to go to closet and try several times before she has stool. There is sensation of weight and pressure in bowels with much rumbling of gas. Abdomen is sensitive in the morning on awakening. Complains of burning, stitching pains in left ovary when constipated. Appetite one time is good, then she may have none at all. She says she cannot get enough to drink; has constant thirst and drinks a great deal of coffee. The mouth and tongue are dry; has feeling as if the skin was peeling from the roof of mouth. Sour taste in mouth all the time; tongue cracked, brown center and red tip.

Does not sleep well; has hard work to get to sleep before midnight and then she wakens frequently with shock in pit of the stomach and a tight suffocating feeling in the chest. Lately she has complained that her heart feels too large for her chest when she walks fast. This oppressive pain is sometimes relieved by belching. For past few weeks face and lips are bluish; has flushes of heat, but only one cheek gets red; the other is pale. For last year her hearing has

6

been failing; she complains of a noise like a tea kettle boiling. There has been scarcely any wax, and what there was would be hard and white. Riding in the cold has always given her earache. She fears to go to bed during this last attack, as she thinks she may die, and she says she dreads to die so much.

There has always been more or less headache, at different times, but the one whch has been the most troublesome is one that begins on the right side of head and goes through to the left until it aches all around. With this there is a drawing in the back of neck and burning pains back of the eyes; some dizziness with sensation as if she were going to fall to the left side. She has an irritable disposition and everything seems to be worse in the morning when she awakens.

Now what is the diagnosis in this case? I do not know. Have never made one. We do not care about the diagnosis, as it is not a disease we wish to treat, but rather this sick woman we are going to try to cure. We have a well-taken case, and from this mass of symptoms we must select some that will individualize this case and make it different from all others. Let us look at the record and see which symptoms we

will select for our repertory analysis. We find
the following general symptoms: Worse after
sleep, thirsty, burning pains, left side and better
during flow. Making a repertory analysis of
these we find under:

Worse after sleep.—*Acon., Apis, Arn., Ars.,
Camp., Carb. s., Carb. v., Caust., Chel., Cocc.,
Con., Euphr., Ferr., Hep.,* LACH., *Lyc., Op.,
Phos. ac., Puls., Rheum, Sabad.,* SEL., *Sep.,
Spong., Staph.,* STRAM., SULPH., *Verat.*

Thirsty.—ACON., *Arn.,* ARS., *Camp., Carb. v.,
Chel., Cocc., Con., Hep., Lach.,* OP., PHOS.,
STRAM., *Sulph.*

Burning pains.—*Acon., Arn.,* ARS., *Carb. v.,
Con., Lach., Op.,* PHOS., SULPH.

Left side.—*Arn.,* LACH., PHOS., SULPH.

Relieved during flow.—LACHESIS.

Here you see we have worked our long case
down to one remedy with five rubrics. We will
now turn to the pathogenesis of *Lachesis* and see
if our selection has been justified. In the *Guid-
ing Symptoms* we find under *Lachesis* not only
the five symptoms we have used, but also each
and every one of the other symptoms; so this
remedy must be homœopathic to the case.

Lachesis, two powders, was sent with the following results: For thirty-six hours after the

administration there was an aggravation of all
the symptoms, which was followed by rapid improvement that has continued ever since   until
the last report, when she wrote that every symptom had disappeared and that she felt as well as
she had ever been in her life.

Let us look at the analysis of constipation, the
great bug-bear of our prescribers, who say
that constipation cannot be affected by the homœopathic remedy. The reason for this statement is that constipation, in the common, *per se,*
cannot be cured, for we have no one remedy for
the disease condition.

Even when we bring our case of constipation
down one step in individualization we are no
better off; taking, for example, constipation with
hard stool, under this common general we find
eighty-three remedies listed under this rubric
(page 635, second edition, Kent); any one of
these remedies might be curative in such a general condition, but if we do not have something
to individualize our case further we are at sea.
Taking character of stool as:

STOOL DRY (page 634).—We narrow our list
to thirty-one remedies, which are as follows:
Æsc., Amm. c., Arg. m., Arg. n., BRY., *Calc. c.,
Cimex., Con., Cupr., Ham., Hep., Kali bi., Kali*

c., *Kali s.*, LAC. D., LYC., *Nat. m.*, NIT. AC., NUX
v., OP., PHOS., *Plat., Plb., Podo., Prun., Sanic.,*
SIL., *Stann., Sulph.*, ZINC.

With this condition is often associated inactivity of rectum, *i. e.*, not having a desire for stool for three or four days.

INACTIVITY OF RECTUM (page 619).—We find fourteen of the above thirty-one remedies, in the first and second grade, which allows us to narrow our group of curative remedies to the following: BRY., *Calc. c.*, KALI C., *Lyc.*, NAT. M., NUX V., OP., PHOS., *Plat.*, PLB., *Podo*, SANIC., SIL., *Sulph.*

The stool may crumble, and if such is the case it will help you to further particularize the above fourteen remedies in order to find the one curative remedy in this individual case.

CRUMBLING (page 634).—This rubric gives us only five of the above fourteen which have crumbling stool, and are as follows: *Nat. m., Op., Plat., Podo., Sulph.*

The best we have been able to do with the symptoms that refer to the constipation, *per se*, has been to narrow down to five remedies, and but one of these five will be curative. You say we might give all five at once in a gun-shot prescription, and that is what some men do, and

then say that Homœopathy will never cure constipation.   Or that you might give first one and
then the other in rotation, but you would never
cure the case that way, although one of these
five remedies will be curative if given alone.   We
must look for other symptoms of the patient, and
you will always be able to find some in every
case that will help us to individualize this patient so we may find the one remedy.

Suppose BURNING PAIN AFTER STOOL (p. 624).
We find that this rubric only contains *Natrum
mur.* and *Sulphur* of the above five remedies.
We are now down to two remedies either one of
which may be curative. . Look at the tongue and
see if you cannot find some symptom there which
will help you out.   Let us suppose that this patient had a heavily coated tongue, but that along
the edges there were spots which were clean.
This would be known as mapped tongue.   Look
under rubric, TONGUE MAPPED IN CIRCLES ON
SIDES (page 411).   We find that of our two
remedies only *Natrum mur.* has this symptom, so
if you have no marked generals to rule out
Natrum mur. it would be the remedy and would
cure the case, unless there was some tissue change
or growth which from pressure was causing an
occlusion of the bowel.   In taking these old

cases of constipation do not expect to give one dose, or a dozen doses, in rapid succession, and expect the constipation to disappear over night or in a week. These cases are usually long standing, they all have the constipation habit, and most of them the cathartic habit, and have to be carried along with your remedies in series, mayhap for several months, before a cure will be established.

In order to cure your case you must insist upon the cathartics being stopped at once, and until your remedy has changed conditions so as to establish a normal stool you must depend upon diet and an enema of warm water to empty the lower bowel.

Form of Case Record.

Mind.—Place all symptoms of mind under this heading, but be sure and leave space on your sheet for symptoms that you may discover at subsequent sittings.

Head.—Here will be placed pains, hair symptoms, movements of head, etc.

Stomach.—This group will include pains, food desires and aversions, eating and drinking, appetite, thirst, nausea, vomiting, eructations and sensations.

Abdomen.—You may place under this heading symptoms referring to constipation, diarrhœa, sensations as pain, pressure, etc., symptoms of urination, defecation, bladder and male genitals.

Menses.—These symptoms are of so much importance to the female case that a separate heading should be made. All symptoms referring to the female generative organs, to child birth, hæmorrhages, etc., may be placed in this group.

Chest.—Symptoms referring to coughs, pains and sensations, expectoration, breathing, heart, pulse, breasts, etc., may be placed under this head.

Back.—Sensations, pains, etc.

Extremities.—All symptoms referring to the upper and lower extremities.

Sleep.—Such symptoms as refer to the condition of sleep, dreams, etc.

Generalities.—Here place all symptoms which refer to conditions or modalities that affect the patient as a whole, not already covered by the mentals.

With the symptoms of your case arranged in this orderly manner, from Mind to Generalities, we have a record to which it is easy to refer and from which it is easy to individualize the record for repertory study.

Part II.

Analysis of Forty Homœopathic Remedies.

These forty remedies will be far from the number required in all your cases, and the forty I have included in my list will contain, no doubt, some which you never use in your individual work, while, on the other hand, some will be lacking which you find of daily use. Any list of so small a proportion of our vast materia medica would necessarily be open to such criticism; but I think that by the arrangement of this list of remedies you will acquire—by giving them a few minutes' study each day—a working knowledge of the remedies you use. If it is possible for me to enable you to systematize these few remedies then I am sure that you will arrange those which you find most often indicated, but which are absent from my list, so that you may then have a working knowledge of the remedies in which you are personally interested.

Consistent use of the repertory leads us to the study of our remedies in a scientific, rational manner, from center to circumference, from the mind to skin, noting the effect of the drug upon the provers, as given in the pathogenesis, in the will, the intellect and responses to every environment, thus learning to observe the disordered patient rather than pathological changes in the organs or parts.

In trying to have an image of a remedy in mind learn to keep an orderly general picture of its action as a whole, following these generalities through the particular manifestations as referred to parts rather than only a few so-called characteristics of the remedy for your daily use. Kent's *Materia Medica* has the remedies so arranged and their pathogenesis is so graphically portrayed that, after reading over a remedy in this book, a picture of the general action of the drug is left with you.

The way I study a remedy and the kind of picture I try to carry in mind, for daily use, are illustrated by the following short study of one of our familiar remedies, *Arnica*.

Arnica.

The red strand running through this remedy is the soreness. A general state of soreness throughout the whole body. The joints become sore, the periosteum is sore, the muscles are sore, and the soreness will continue until stiffness begins and we find the sore, stiff rheumatic pains of the *Arnica* patient. The soreness is manifest in the skin, so that there are black and blue marks. The soreness is so marked that pressure is painful and the parts lain on are sore, so sore that he wants to move, to change position frequently, for the longer he lies on a part the more sore and sensitive it becomes. He is stiff, so the motion is painful; still the bed is so hard, the parts so sore, that he must move. Therefore, when we see our *Arnica* patient we must expect to find this soreness; if not, *Arnica* will not be the remedy.

There is a general relaxation of the blood vessels in our *Arnica* patients, and this is manifest in the hæmorrhages from various organs. In the subcutaneous tissues this is represented by extravasation of blood under the skin which results in black and blue spots. The *Arnica* state which is associated with or preceding many acute diseases is manifest by this weakened state of the blood vessels, and the patient will wonder how she got so many black and blue marks; even the slightest bruise or pressure will result in this discoloration. Little injuries produce bleeding. On mucous surfaces these result in hæmorrhages. Hæmorrhages of bright red blood which soon clots. The blood of the *Arnica* state soon clots, as is manifest by the blood-streaked or -flecked sputa which will contain many tiny clots.

Arnica developed in its provers violent chills and fever; the fevers are a low, slow form that is associated with inflammation. From the results of the relaxed condition of the blood vessels all the organs of the body are prone to inflammations and hæmorrhages; but with these hæmorrhages we will have this general condition of soreness.

With these conditions we have pains, and the general characteristic pains that call for *Arnica* are, crawling, pricking or paralytic pains as if joints were dislocated. Unsettled pains which shift from one part to another; tingling and tearing pains. With all these conditions are the bruised, sore sensations, and a deep, profound disturbance of the economy which is manifest by weakness; great and profound prostration, fatigue and sleepiness. The countenance in these profound cases will be flushed and dark; there will be a besotted look, as if he was intoxicated, and he speaks and thinks with difficulty. Many cases of cerebral hæmorrhage and the low forms of typhoid will present this typical *Arnica* picture, and unless these patients receive this remedy they will die. From this you will be led to look for *Arnica* in your septic conditions, and it has many symptoms which correspond to septic processes, such as are associated with typhoid and scarlet fever and other low forms of diseases. In septic diseases of every sort we find our patients running into *Arnica* conditions. Surgical septicæmia and blood changes due to surgical shock. Where *Arnica* covers the condition of your patient it will do more to restore the antibacterial power of the blood than any number of vaccines. *Arnica* represents the surgical septic condition more closely than that of the puerperal type. (This latter condition corresponds more closely to *Sulphur*.) Wonderful is its action in preventing suppuration. A severe inflammation will be set up by an injury, a severe bruise upon the muscles, there will follow the pain and soreness and induration with final suppuration. A dose of *Arnica* in the beginning will prevent all this and quickly restore the part to normal.

Bruises. This name at once makes you think of *Arnica,* and for this condition it has been applied externally by all schools and by all people. The external application is better than nothing, but the administration internally is best of all. It is not the bruise, *per se,* that we can expect to relieve; that has happened and cannot be undone, but it is the resulting effects of the bruise

that we wish to prevent and remove, and this
came from the center from the internal structure
and can best be overcome from the center by the
internal action of the remedy.

Injuries to the head, with the resulting nerve
and brain symptoms, send the patient into an
Arnica state, and they will need this remedy to
bring about order no matter how long ago the
injury took place. The resulting shock of surgical operations calls for *Arnica*, and this remedy
is given in routine practice by the surgeons of
our school. The symptoms following operations,
which *Arnica* will remove, are those which are
produced by handling and bruising of the soft
tissues and no others. That is the reason the results are so often disappointing. Those sharp,
cutting pains, the results of the needle or the
knife, will never be removed by *Arnica*, but are
rapidly dispersed by *Staphisagria*. Cuts and
open wounds never call for *Arnica*, only as there
are shock, bruises and contusions.

Thus we have outlined the general action of
our remedy, and these general conditions are always present in a greater or less degree in
every case that calls for *Arnica*. Where there is
no soreness never think of *Arnica*.

The mental symptoms of *Arnica* are striking,

and many of them are symptoms which you would expect to result from shock. Fear, excitement, emotion and horror stand out prominently. The fear that something awful is going to happen, that he is going to die instantly. This is marked and the patient has a horror of death and of the unexpected. In many of the acute conditions we have an obstinate and irritable patient. He will want to fight with you and to drive you from the room. This excessive irritability will often be followed by a delirium. Indifference, anxiety and hopelessness run through the mental state. In the low states we find a stupor. He is hard to arouse, and when you do wake him he will be confused and will not know where he is. Mental exertion, motion or physical exertion, all aggravate his condition.

The pains in the head are pressive, cramplike, darting and tingling, and are made worse by walking, ascending and mental exertion. There is nothing very distinctive about the particular symptoms of the head, but any pains or conditions that arise from injuries will lead one to think of *Arnica*.

There is a peculiar symptom under this remedy which is associated with the eyes. He must keep his eyes open. They come open spontaneously, he cannot hold them closed himself. As soon as the eyes are closed he gets dizzy, things go round and it makes him sick.

The pains of the nose are sore pains, as if bruised; much nosebleed when first blowing nose in the morning. The coryza of *Arnica* comes in the evening when going to sleep, but with this will be the general bruised condition, the soreness that will differentiate it from *Nux* or *Pulsatilla.*

One of the keynotes of *Arnica* is manifest in the face; heat and redness of the face with coldness of the body. It seems as if the blood had left the body and gone to the head. The expression of the face is peculiar. We have a deep mahogany redness, with an intoxicated, besotted look; he looks as if his mental condition was benumbed; looks as if he was making an effort to find the right thing to say or do but cannot. He is stupid and he looks it. In injuries about the face, especially about the eye and cheek bones, where the periosteum seems to have been injured, we find that *Arnica* will remove the first effects, the superficial soreness, the black and blue condition; but after this has been done away with there will remain a soreness that appears to be in the bone itself. We could give *Arnica* indefinitely, and these symptoms would not disappear, but *Hypericum* will follow and remove them speedily.

The general condition of *Arnica* is exhibited in the mouth by soreness of the teeth. Soreness at the roots of the teeth, as if they were being pressed out. The gums bleed easily. Hæmorrhages from the gums after extraction of the teeth. This is one of our leaders in bleeders after teeth extraction. Soreness of the gums after extraction. This remedy will do more to remove the soreness from the gums after extraction than all the mouth washes you ever heard of. (Sepia is another remedy which is useful in this condition, especially in the nervous women who have been made sick by having a few teeth extracted.) The mouth tastes bitter and like rotten eggs. This is from the eructations, which are bitter and have the odor of spoiled eggs; this taste remains in the mouth and you can almost smell it on the breath; therefore, the books give "putrid smell from the mouth;" this as well as the eructations are worse in the morning. These eructations burn as they come up and cause a burning from the stomach to the fauces.

With this large amount of gas in the stomach we have a loss of appetite. A loathing of food;

7

even the sight of food is repulsive and nauseates. Meat, milk and broth are especially repugnant, and even his tobacco nauseates. Aversion to tobacco, to even the smell of tobacco smoke, stands high in this remedy. (What does a peculiar symptom like this mean and what weight shall we place on it. We cannot expect to give all the ladies and others to whom tobacco may be offensive a dose or two of *Arnica* and make them lovers of the weed, but where a man has become a user of the weed, where the habit has become fixed so that his tobacco is a necessity, and then have some disturbance of his economy so effect him that what he desired and craved he now dislikes, and has such an aversion to it that the odor is even nauseating, we have what we are justified in calling a peculiar condition, and when this arises we will give it a prominent place in our symptom picture.)

The generals are still with us when we study the effects of *Arnica* on the stomach. The sore, aching extending through to back. The stomach is so sore it feels as if it rubbed the spine, and as if the spine was made sore by this pressure. Pressing pains in the stomach; as if it was pressed by the hand. This pressure continues until it seems to rise to the neck; then he feels nauseated and bitter water comes into the mouth. The stomach is so sore that everything seems to press against it as if the xiphoïd process was pressed inward; as if a weight was on or in the stomach; as if a stone laid in the stomach. Nausea; retching; ineffectual retching; they retch and retch and try to vomit, and after straining for some time they vomit blood and bloody mucus. The blood will be dark and coagulated. After this the stomach will be more sore and burn.

Inflammation of the liver and spleen often take on *Arnica* symptoms. Shooting and stitches in the spleen and pressure as if from a stone in the liver are found under this remedy; with this condition we have a distended tympanitic abdomen with passage of much foul flatus smelling like rotten eggs. The soreness and bruised sensation are stronger in all the abdominal symptoms.

With a condition in the stomach and bowels which led to the above symptoms you would expect to have trouble with the stools; you would look for a diarrhœa, and under *Arnica* we find slimy, mucus stools; brown, fermented, like yeast; undigested; bloody; purulent; dark, bloody mucus; large fetid, fæcal; yellow, offensive and sour.

A peculiar stool symptom of *Arnica* is the involuntary stool during sleep. The rumbling and colic in the abdomen are relieved after stool. Another of the peculiar symptoms of this remedy is that the diarrhœa is aggravated, as well as the accompanying bowel symptoms, by lying on the left side. During the stool there is urging, tenesmus, sore bruised pain in abdomen; cutting in intestines; rumbling and pressure in abdomen. Tenesmus in rectum and bladder. After stool they are weak and prostrated and are obliged to lie down.

From the low state that the *Arnica* patient represents we would look for its counterpart in typhoid, where its general soreness and weakness resemble *Baptisia*, *Pyrogen* and *Rhus;* but where the general and characteristic symptoms of *Arnica* are present it will be curative in cases where vaccines and other remedies will fail.

The peculiar urine of *Arnica* is dark brown, with brick dust sediment; the urine is full of urates and uric acid that we find associated with rheumatic cases. From the general relaxed condition of the blood vessels we get bloody urine, hæmorrhages from the bladder. "Urination involuntary when running" is peculiar to *Arnica*.

The symptoms of *Arnica* referring to the

female sexual organs are distinctive; here we find the character of the hæmorrhage changed to a bright red flow mixed with clots. The flow feels hot as it passes the vulva. Menses are profuse, especially after a blow, a fall or a shock to the system. The general soreness is marked, and the pelvis is so sore it prevents her from walking erect. The uterus is sensitive, bleeds easily; discharges of blood between periods, with nausea. Bleeding after coition. *Arnica* is especially useful in nervous women who cannot stand pain.

Not only for the resulting shock and effects of the bruising resulting from labor is *Arnica* useful, but it has a field of usefulness in changing the character of the labor pains. These pains in your *Arnica* patient will be too feeble and irregular, resulting from fatigue of the muscular tissue. They do nothing, although so severe that they drive her to distraction. Feels sore and must often change her position. Vagina sore and sensitive so she does not want to be examined. Great soreness of the back during labor. *Arnica* high will often prevent after-pains. It will contract the blood vessels and prevent post-partum hæmorrhages. Used in routine practice it does much to relieve the distressing after symptoms, both mental and physical, of labor.

The cough of *Arnica* is dry and is caused from tickling in larynx and trachea; the cough is worse evening until midnight, from motion, warm room and after drinking. The expectoration is scanty, difficult, of glairy mucus mixed with tiny clots of dark blood. The general soreness of the remedy is marked in the chest and is shown in whooping cough where the child will cry before the paroxysm. The coughing causes blood-shot eyes, nosebleed and expectoration of foaming blood. With the cough is a burning rawness of the chest, stitches in left chest, which are worse from motion and pressure.

From the general soreness and bruised sensations in the muscles you would be led to think of your *Arnica* patient as a rheumatic patient, and such is the case. *Arnica* is full of bruised, paralytic, sore and stiff rheumatic pains. The joints ache and feel as if they were bruised. The soreness is so marked that the *Arnica* patient is full of fear; afraid he will be touched; afraid of jars; doesn't want you to come near for fear you will touch and hurt the sore joint or muscle. In the back we have violent pains in the spine, sore pains; spine feels as if it would not hold the weight of the body. Small of the back feels as if it had been beaten. Pressive pain between the scapulæ.

The rheumatic pains in the extremities are associated with heaviness. The legs are so heavy that it seems as if he could not lift them; this heaviness is due to the paralytic pains in the joints, and is constant both when at rest and in motion. Limbs are sensitive to concussions, as the jar of carriage or of walking. In the arms we have violent twitchings going from the shoulder to joints of middle finger. Crackings in wrist joints, worse in right, as if dislocated; drawing pains in wrist relieved by letting hand hang down. Pressing, tearing pains in fingers. Cramps in fingers of left hand. These tearing and drawing pains as if sprained are also found in the lower extremities. The hips feel as if sprained, with a pressive drawing in the left hip, which is worse from extending the thigh when sitting. The tearing pain on right external malleolus and on dorsum of foot with drawing in outer half of foot is peculiar to *Arnica*. Gout in joint of great toe with redness; pain worse towards evening and from pressure. These pains as if bruised and sprained with discoloration are a picture of sprains and here the remedy administered internally will take the soreness and discoloration from the sprained ankle and remove the first effects of the sprain; those symptoms which remain after *Arnica* are usually amenable to *Ruta* and *Rhus*.

The most severe action of the remedy on the nerves is the paralysis, the prostration, the general weakness and sinking of strength; so weak he can scarcely move a limb. The prostration and general sinking of strength corresponds to the low state found in typhoid and other zymotic fevers.

The *Arnica* patient has many symptoms during sleep, those symptoms which resemble the stupor of apoplexy and the sleep symptoms of meningitis find their counterpart in *Arnica*. One of the peculiar sleep symptoms is that the patient will be sleepy all day but cannot sleep at night.

Your *Arnica* patient is full of chills; chilly, with heat and redness of one check; head hot, body cold; internal chill with external heat; thirst during chill (resembling *Eupatorium*), he will drink and drink, becoming more chilly all the time, and will have the characteristic stomach symptoms, and finally vomit a bitter, sour fluid. Chilly on only one side of body, and

that of the side lain upon. Many of the intermittent symptoms closely resemble *Eupatorium*,
but the general and stomach symptoms will allow
you to differentiate in this disease.

Remember the generals of this remedy and you
will find its greatest usefulness after mechanical
injuries, no matter what disease name you may
give to the condition arising from this source.
Arnica will help not only to remove the disease
condition, but if given early will prevent many
of the resultant symptoms of shock from appearing. Most of the particular symptoms of
this remedy can be figured out by applying the
general state of the remedy to all organs or
parts of the body. Keep these in mind and you
will see how often many symptoms or disease
conditions can be removed by this remedy alone;
given internally and without recourse to any
adjuvants. If it has the generals of *Arnica* it is
an *Arnica* case, and does not require *Baptisia*,
Bryonia, *Rhus* or anything else to be curative.

Suggestions as to Method of Study and Use of the Following Analysis.

Take first the twenty-two rubrics and memo-
rize the group of remedies found under each
one, paying attention first to the generals. After
you have become familiar with your list of rem-

edies then learn the particular circumstance of the remedy under each rubric. This will give you a ground work of these remedies that will be of use to you in the daily work of prescribing for your acute cases. After you have become familiar with the above symptoms you may broaden your knowledge of each remedy by reference to the materia medica. It has been my experience (as well as that of my students) that a few minutes' study each day will soon give you a comprehensive knowledge of the remedies that will be in shape to use at the bedside.

Take, for example, a cold patient, one who is shivering with the cold, and, although covered by blankets, cannot get warm. We find this patient having burning pains; he may be thirsty or not, there may be œdema of mucous membrane with stinging pains. There may be scanty urine or any number of symptoms referring to a particular organ or to disease condition, which might lead you to think of *Apis*, but the fact that your patient was cold would rule that remedy out and turn your thoughts to a remedy found under the first rubric, *Cold and aggravation from cold*. Here you would find that one of the twenty-six remedies given would be one which would be homœopathic to the patient in hand.

Take another example of a patient with throbbing pains. The first thought of the majority of our men when they hear throbbing pains mentioned is *Belladonna;* but fourteen remedies in our list of forty have throbbing pains, and *Aconite, Calcarea carb., Phosphorus, Pulsatilla* and *Sepia* all have this characteristic pain in a higher degree than overworked *Belladonna.* We will know at least from this analysis that one of our fourteen remedies will be indicated, but must individualize more closely to find the one remedy. If the patient who exhibits the throbbing pains is worse after midnight think of those remedies that have an aggravation after midnight, and we will at once see that among these ten we have *Bry., Calc. c., Phos., Sulph.* and *Sil.* Here we have five, any one of which may be the remedy to help your patient's throbbing pains. We learn that the patient is chilly, that the pains are worse from warmth, but that she desires very cold drinks. This at once lets us know that *Phosphorus* alone of the above remedies will be the one which the patient requires.

Many other examples could be cited as to the use of the preceding scheme, but to those who will look to this work for assistance they would not be necessary, and the student who begins to get a useable knowledge of our materia medica from this analysis will find that his learning of the remedies by this method will enable him to discriminate, individualize and differentiate his remedy and patient quickly, accurately and with an ease which will astonish him.

Forty Remedies.

The following remedies are those we will analyze: *Aconite; Arnica; Arsenicum; Apis; Antimonium tart.; Belladonna; Bryonia; Calcarea. carb.; Carbo veg.; Causticum; China; Chamomilla; Colocynth; Digitalis; Drosera; Dulcamara; Gelsemium; Graphites; Hepar; Hyoscyamus; Ignatia; Ipecac; Lachesis; Lycopodium; Mercurius; Natrum mur.; Nitric ac.; Nux vom.; Phosphorus; Phosphoric ac.; Podophyllum; Rhus tox.; Sulphur; Sepia; Silicea; Staphisagria; Thuja; Veratrum alb.* and *Zincum.*

In order that we may analyze these remedies I have taken twenty-two rubrics which cover the generals as to: (1) Heat and cold; (2) mental states as related to (a) restlessness, (b) fear, (c) crossness and irritability, and (d) tearfulness; the modalities as to (3) motion, and (4) position when lying; (5) the time of aggravation as to (a) afternoon, (b) after midnight, and

(c) after sleep; aggravation and amelioration from (6) pressure; generals and particulars as related to (7) thirst; aggravation from (8) eating and (9) drinking; (10) the character of the pain as found under (a) burning, (b) cutting, (c) sore, (d) throbbing, (e) cramping, and (f) bursting.

I believe that with the right use of these twenty-two rubrics we can eliminate remedies, in the majority of our acute cases, so that we may arrive at the one and only one which will cover our individual case.

Taking our first rubric,

Cold and Aggravation from Cold.

This is covered by the following twenty-six of our forty remedies, either in the first or second degree: *Acon.;* ARS.; *Bell.; Bry.;* CALC. c.; CHINA; *Carbo veg.;* CAUST.; *Coloc.;* DULC.; GRAPH.; HEP.; *Ipec.; Ign.; Lach.; Lyc.; Merc.;* · NUX v.; *Nat. ac.;* PHOS.; PHOS. AC.; RHUS; SEP.; *Sulph.;* SIL.

In using this rubric we must distinguish between coldness, which is a lack of vital heat, and an aggravation from cold in various forms, or amelioration from heat. These are two distinct phases. A patient who craves warmth and cannot keep warm is cold, but the particular symptoms may be aggravated from warmth and ameliorated from cold. An example is seen in *Phosphorus,* which is a very cold patient, but his stomach symptoms are better from cold drinks. When he is sick he craves cold drinks, which, however, are vomited as soon as they become warm in the stomach. His head symptoms are also better from cold. *Lycopodium,* on the other hand, is a warm remedy and often cannot stand heat, but his stomach symptoms are ameliorated by hot food and drink. *Arsenicum* is a very cold remedy, yet his head symptoms are relieved by cold.

Looking to the particular circumstances under which each of the remedies are affected by cold your leaders will be:

Arsenicum when patient is cold and has general aggravation from cold, except the headache, which will be relieved by cold.

Calcarea carb. has chilliness with aversion to open air and sensitiveness to cold, damp air, with aggravation of pains from slightest draft.

China, where there is chilliness with coldness of internal parts.

Causticum, where there is coldness that warmth does not relieve. The cough, diarrhœa, and rheumatism are worse from cold; paralysis from cold.

Dulcamara, complaints brought on by cold, damp weather and living in damp places; coryza, cough and neuralgia are worse from cold.

Graphites, predominantly chilly; the coryza, bone pains and stomach are worse from cold, while the skin symptoms are worse from warmth.

Hepar is another chilly patient; extremely sensitive to slight draft; is worse from cold wind and cold drinks; aggravation from getting a part cold.

Lycopodium, while a warm remedy, stands high in its particulars, being aggravated by cold, as its stomach, cough, throat and headache.

Nitric acid, where there is icy coldness and aggravation from least exposure; soles of feet cold. The coryza and chilblains worse, but cough better from cold.

Nux vomica has general chilliness over whole body; sensitive to open air; aversion to uncovering. Cough and headache are made worse.

Phosphorus is very cold, with coldness locally in the cerebellum, stomach, hands and feet; neuralgia, rheumatism, cough and diarrhœa are worse from cold, while the stomach and head symptoms are relieved by cold.

Phosphoric acid, where there is sensitiveness to drafts; abdomen and one side of face is cold.

Rhus tox., where there is internal chilliness; aggravation from cold, wet, open air, drafts, cold drinks and cold east wind.

Silica, where there is general chilliness, always cold; cold weather, cold water and cold in general aggravate.

—

If the above do not cover your case examine the following:

Aconite, is worse from cold, dry winds, complaints from riding in; makes the coryza, conjunctivitis, toothache, croup, cough and rheumatism worse.

Belladonna, where there is aggravation by going from warm to cold; aggravation from drafts and cold wind.

Bryonia, where there is chilliness; complaints from cold drinks in hot weather.

Carbo veg., where there is susceptibility to cold. Cold nose, knees, etc.

Colocynth, where there is coldness of whole body; aggravation from cold weather; stomach, coryza, gastritis and rheumatism are worse from cold; tearing, stinging pain in face from taking cold.

Ipecac has oversensitiveness to both heat and cold; colic from cold drinks; aggravation in winter.

Ignatia has chill predominating; cold winds and air alike aggravate; washing hands in cold water aggravates pains; nose, feet, and legs up to knees are cold.

Lachesis has a coldness over the whole body; limbs and upper lip cold; throat worse from drafts.

Mercurius, cannot bear cold; extremely sensitive. Coldness in ears, testicles and lower limbs.

Natrum mur., icy coldness about the heart; coldness of feet, joints, back and stomach.

Sepia has coldness over whole body; sensitive to cold, damp air; the cough, eruptions, toothache and rheumatism are worse from cold.

Sulphur is worse in cold, windy weather; in damp, cold weather; the throat and the diarrhœa are worse from cold.

Warmth and Aggravation from Warmth.

Are covered by the following eighteen remedies: APIS; *Ant. t.; Bry.; Dulc.; Dros.; Graph.; Ipec.; Lach., Lyc., Merc., Nat. mur.; Phos.,* PULS.; *Secale; Sulph.; Sepia; Verat.* and *Zinc.*

Your leaders will be:

Apis, where there is general condition of warmth with aggravation from warm room. The chill and headache are worse from warmth.

8

Pulsatilla is too warm, with great internal heat; aggravation from warm room and warm food; from heat of stove, with general aggravation of all complaints from heat.

Secale, cannot bear heat, will throw off all covering; aversion to heat; internal pains much aggravated by heat. Warm drinks aggravate the coldness of stomach.

—

Antimonium tart., the head is worse from warmth; cough is worse from warm drinks; aggravation from getting warm in bed; drowsy from warmth.

Bryonia, head, face and chills are worse. Cough worse from warm air and room.

Drosera, while always chilly, has < of cough; ulcers, and pain in long bones from warmth.

Dulcamara, the cough, nettle rash and sneezing worse from warmth.

Graphites, is worse from dry heat in the evening and night; itching is worse from heat of stove; toothache is worse from warmth.

Ipecac, the heat aggravates the chill; worse from warm, moist, south winds.

Lachesis, worse in warm spring weather (*e. g.*, diarrhœa) and from warmth of bed; diarrhœa aggravated.

Lycopodium has desire for open air; warmth
< eruptions; warm room < cough and head-
ache. Aversion to warm food [warm drinks >
pain in throat]; longs for cold food although it
< diarrhœa and cough.

Mercurius, the external pains worse from
warmth of bed; extremely sensitive to heat;
headache, mumps, toothache, rheumatic pains
and itching are worse.

Natrum mur., is worse from heat of sun and
in summer; cough and headache worse; toothache aggravated from warm food.

Phosphorus, while cold, cannot tolerate heat
near back; warm water causes toothache; warm
food causes diarrhœa; warm drinks < cough;
stomach is worse from heat; hands, face and
arms become red from heat, and itching is worse.

Sepia, general aggravation in warm room,
warm climate, and from covering; conjunctivitis
and headache worse; breathing oppressed from
warmth.

Sulphur. Too warm. Throws off covers;
< warm room, warmth of bed and heat of sun;
headache, burning of feet and itching especially
<.

Veratrum has cough worse in warm room;
neuralgia worse from warmth of bed; diarrhœa
worse in warm weather.

Zincum, complaints from becoming heated and getting cold; rheumatism from overheating; warm room aggravates headache.

Restlessness.

The following thirty-two remedies have restlessness, either mental or physical: Acon.; Ars.; *Apis; Ant. t.;* Bell.; *China;* Calc. c.; *Carbo v.; Caust.; Cham.;* Coloc.; *Dulc.;* Dig.; Hyos.; *Ipec.; Ign.;* Lyc.; *Lach.;* Merc.; *Nux v.; Nat. mur.; Nit. ac.; Phos. ac.;* Puls.; *Rhus t.;* Sulph.; Secale; Sep.; Sil.; Staph.; *Thuj.;* Verat. A.

Your leaders will be:

Aconite changes position constantly; impatient and anxious at night; must walk or move about, although it does not relieve pain. Does everything in great haste.

Arsenicum, mental and physical restlessness; goes from one bed to another.

Belladonna, during colic; with cardiac trouble; striking, biting; wants to fly away from pains.

Calcarea carb., mental anxiety and restlessness; child cross, fretful and restless.

Digitalis, where restlessness is associated with great nervous weakness.

Hyoscyamus, turns from one place to another.

Lycopodium, restless from oversensitiveness to pain; during colic.

Mercurius, mental; desire to flee, with anxiety; everything is done hastily; must constantly change places; uneasiness; restless 8 P. M. until morning.

Pulsatilla, mental restlessness and change-ability forces him to get up at night; cannot rest, although motion aggravates.

Rhus tox., cannot remain quiet although it hurts to move; mental restlessness.

Secale, spasmodic twitchings with irregular movements of whole body; arms in constant motion; head jerks about from side to side.

Sepia, throbbing in all the limbs will not permit of quiet.

Silica, fidgety; starts at least noise; internal restlessness and excitement; body restless when sitting long.

Staphisagria, restlessness with lack of inclination to move; hurts to move.

Sulphur, uneasiness and excitation of nervous system; constantly moving feet.

Zincum, feet fidgety; must move them constantly.

—

The following have restlessness in the second degree:

Apis, is very busy; does nothing right; changes

kind of work frequently; uneasiness, mental and physical.

Antimonium tart., anxiety; tossing about; throws arms.

Carbo veg., restless at night, or 4 to 6 P. M.; mental restlessness.

Causticum, restlessness of body, worse evening; wants to run away; obliged to walk about.

Chamomilla, child quiet only when carried; kicks when carried; whining restlessness; tosses about in bed; great restlessness with anxiety and impatience; jerking and twitching in sleep.

China, compelled to jump out of bed.

Colocynth, restlessness with diarrhœa; weak but has to move; finds rest in no position; headache compels him to walk.

Dulcamara, great restlessness; impatience; general uneasiness.

Ignatia, trembling of hands when writing; change of position often relieves pains; jerkings and twitchings in various parts of muscles.

Ipecac, is restless in fevers.

Lachesis, must change position frequently, with pain in back and limbs.

Natrum mur., restless with chill; must move limbs constantly; hastiness.

Nitric acid. Restlessness of limbs in evening; twitchings in upper part of body.

Nux vom., great reflex excitability; convulsive twitchings of single muscles; body tossed to right side and back again; legs drawn up to body with sudden jerk, then forcibly thrust out again.

Phosphoric acid, walking relieves oppression of chest, pain in loins, hip joints, thighs, and pain in the bones.

Thuja, tossing about at night from anxiety; mental restlessness.

Veratrum, must walk about; mental restlessness; constant twitches and silly motions; cannot dress herself.

Irritability

The following thirty-four remedies are cross and irritable:

ACON.; *Arn.; Ars.;* APIS; *Ant. t.,* BELL.; BRY.; CHAM.; CALC. c.; *China;* CARBO V.; CAUST.; *Coloc.; Dulc.; Dig.; Gels.;* HEP.; *Lach.;* LYC.; *Merc.;* NUX V.; NAT. MUR.; NIT. AC.; PHOS.; PHOS. AC.; PULS.; RHUS T.; SULPH.; SEP.; SIL.; *Staph.; Thuj.; Verat.;* ZINC.

Your leaders will be:

Aconite, pains intolerable, drive him crazy; ailments from anger.

Apis, is hard to please; irritable; ailments from rage and vexation.

Arsenicum, peevish, waspish and quarrelsome.

Belladonna, quarrelsome; violent rage; bites and strikes and screams.

Bryonia, weeping; angry; peevish; wants to be alone.

Calcarea carb., is cross during day; obstinate; vindictive; easily angered.

Carbo veg., is excitable and peevish; strikes, kicks and bites in rage.

Causticum, is peevish, fretful, quarrelsome, disturbed and ill-humored.

Chamomilla is always out of humor; peevish; quarrelsome; angry.

Hepar, gets angry at least trifle; obstinate; cross; extreme violence; threatens murder and arson; passionate fretfulness.

Lycopodium, is peevish and cross on awaking; cannot endure least opposition; obstinate; defiant, arbitrary; morose, worse before menses.

Nux vom., is sullen; quarrelsome; oversensitive; scolding; ill-humor; gets so mad he cries; stomach complaints after anger; frightened easily.

Natrum mur., ill-humor in the morning; great irritability; cross when spoken to; gets into passion about trifles; bad effects from anger or reserved displeasure.

Nitric acid, is headstrong; trembles while quarreling; fits of rage with cursing; vexed at trifles; sad and obstinate.

Phosphorus, is excitable and easily angered; irritability of mind and body; prostrated from least unpleasant impression.

Phosphoric acid has a condition of silent peevishness and aversion to conversation.

Pulsatilla, is out of sorts with everything; fretful, easily enraged; taciturn.

Rhus tox., impatient; vexed at every trifle; depressed and ill-humored.

Sepia, vexed and disposed to scold; fretful about business; irritability alternating with indifference; nervous irritability.

Silica, headstrong; obstinate and violent.

Sulphur is obstinate; destructive and easily excited.

Thuja is easily angered about trifles; obstinate and quarrelsome.

Zincum is cross towards evening; irritable; peevish; terrified; fretful; cries when vexed.

The following remedies will be less often of use:

Antimonium tart. is worse after anger; weeps and cries in anger.

Arnica is oversensitive; ailments from anger.

China, taciturn; ill-humor increased by petting and caressing; stubborn and disobedient.

Colocynth, throws things in anger; diarrhœa, vomiting and suppressed menses from anger.

Dulcamara, is easily angered and quarrelsome.

Digitalis, is gloomy and disturbed.

Gelsemium, is gloomy and wants to be left alone.

Lachesis, has a sensitive and jealous disposition.

Mercurius, has desire to kill person contradicting her. Taciturn.

Staphisagria, has ailments from vexation or reserved displeasure; child cries for things, which, when it gets it, throws away.

Veratrum alb., curses and howls all night; attacks of rage with swearing.

Fear.

ACON.; *Arn.; Ars.; Bell.; Bry.; Calc. c.; Caust.; Carbo v.;* DIG.; *Gels.;* GRAPH.; *Hep.; Hyos.;* IGN.; LYC.; *Merc.; Nat. m.; Nux v.;* PHOS.; *Puls.; Sulph.; Verat.*

Among these twenty-two remedies you will find your leaders to be:

Aconite, has ailments from fright; afraid of crowds; ghosts; death; dark; of falling; to cross a street.

Belladonna, has fear, worse in day time; of ghosts; of water; hides from fear.

Digitalis, is constantly tortured by fear of death; fear of future.

Graphites, is apprehensive; full of fear in the morning.

Ignatia, has a dread of every trifle; terror; fear of thieves.

Lycopodium, is timid; apprehensive; easily frightened even by slight noises.

Phosphorus, has a fear and dread of death; fear during thunder storms; of faces, as if horrible faces were looking out of every corner.

——

The following remedies also may be found useful:

Arnica, has fear of being struck or even touched; of death.

Arsenicum, has great fear, anxiety with restlessness and prostration. Fear and dread of death; of being left alone.

Bryonia, apprehensive; dread of future; anxiety about and fear of death.

Calcarea carb., fears imaginary things that happen to her; anxiety about recovery; that she will become insane. Fear of death; of consumption; of being alone (evenings).

Carbo veg., is easily frightened and has nightly fear of ghosts.

Causticum is timorous, is afraid to go to bed alone; full of frightful ideas; that something unpleasant will happen; fear of death.

Gelsemium, has lack of courage; fear of death; bad effects of fright.

Hepar, has violent fright on going to sleep.

Hyoscyamus, stands high in complaints from fright; fear of being alone, of being injured, and of poison.

Mercurius, is afraid that she will kill herself; of being alone; that he will lose his mind.

Natrum mur., fears that foetus will be marked; that something is going to happen; that she will lose her reason; chorea after fright.

Nux vom., inclined to commit suicide, but is afraid to die; frightened easily; anxious about condition; terrifying illusions.

Pulsatilla, has diarrhœa after fright; dread of people.

Sulphur, has a fear that he will be ruined financially.

Veratrum alb., has a fear that takes breath away; coldness, fainting and involuntary stool after fright; of death; easily frightened.

Tearfulness.

Patients that are tearful are covered by the following twenty remedies:

Acon.; APIS; *Ant. t.; Bell; Bry.; Calc. c.; Carbo v.;* CAUST.; *Dig.;* GRAPH.; *Hep.;* IGN.; LYCO.; NAT. M.; *Phos.;* PULS.; RHUS T.; SULPH.; SEP.; VERAT.

Your leaders will be:

Apis, when they are discouraged and despondent.

Calcarea carb., when they are easily offended. Despair of life.

Causticum, is hopeless, looks on dark side of everything; weeps during day; whines; least thing makes child cry.

Graphites, has inclination to weep; cries about slightest occurrence; weeps from music.

Ignatia, has inward grief; alternating weeping and laughter; sits alone and weeps.

Lycopodium, cries all day; weeps when thanked; sensitive and melancholy.

Natrum mur., is sad and weeps without cause; when spoken to; concern about future.

Phosphorus, sadness regularly occurring at twilight; prostrated from least unpleasant impression; tearfulness alternating with mirth.

Pulsatilla, cries from sadness or joy; from

vexation and mortification; over nothing; when
telling her symptoms.

Rhus tox., has weeping with prostration, worse
evening; desires solitude; begins to weep without
knowing why.

Sepia, has involuntary weeping; great sadness
with frequent attacks of weeping; worse walking in open air.

Sulphur, cries from consolation; during day
and because she is depressed about illness.

Veratrum alb., cries, howls and curses over
fancied misfortunes.

Less often indicated will be:

Aconite, sadness alternating with laughter.

Antimonium tart., cries from anger; from being touched; during cough; whines.

Belladonna, howls; cries from vexation and
hopelessness.

Carbo veg., thinks he has committed some
crime, which causes him to weep.

Digitalis, sighing and weeping; worse from
music; tearfulness with low spirits.

Hepar, is low spirited and sad, must cry for
hours.

Aggravation from Lying.

Aggravation from lying is covered by seventeen remedies, as follows:

Acon.; ARS.; APIS; *Ant. t.; Bell.;* CHAM.; DULC., DROS., HYOS., *Lach.,* LYC., *Nux v.,* PHOS.; *Phos. ac.;* PULS.; RHUS T.; SEP.

Your leaders will be:

Arsenicum, must lie but pains are worse; breathing is worse.

Apis, worse from lying on left side; chest, breathing and cough are worse lying on left side.

Chamomilla, flickering before eyes, nausea, vertigo, neuralgia, pain in thighs, and swallowing are worse; aggravation from lying on back.

Dulcamara, has headache, cough and rheumatic pains worse when lying.

Drosera, is worse from lying in bed; on the sore side; aggravation of cough.

Hyoscyamus, lies on back, but cough is worse when lying.

Lycopodium, the cough is worse from lying on left, and better on right side; lying on back aggravates breathing; abdomen and cough worse lying on right side.

Phosphorus, lying on back relieves pneumonia; on right side relieves diarrhœa, stitches in chest and after pneumonia. Lying on left side aggravates heart, cough, rheumatism, and diarrhœa.

Pulsatilla, is worse from lying on back during

pains, and from lying on the left or painless side. Urging to urinate aggravated lying on back.

Rhus tox., lying aggravates the cough; vertigo; back; rheumatism and trembling.

—

When the above do not cover the case one of the following may be indicated:

Aconite, lying is unbearable during fever; palpitation worse; chest and cough aggravated from lying on right side. Cheek lain on sweats.

Antimonium tart., is worse from lying on affected side; earache; vomits when lying any way but on right side.

Belladonna, headache and cough are aggravated lying on right side; aggravates pain in liver.

Lachesis, has pain in lungs, left arm, back, in spine, and suffocation, all worse lying; involuntary urination when lying.

Nux vom., cough and pains in chest worse lying on back; cannot lie on right side; asthma; sneezing and headache worse lying.

Phosphoric acid, vertigo and tickling in chest when lying in bed.

Sepia, headache worse lying on back; lying on left side aggravates cough.

Aggravation from Motion.

The following twenty remedies are worse from motion:

Arn.; Ars.; Apis; BELL.; BRY.; *Carbo v.;* COLOC.; *Dig.; Gels.; Hep.; Ipec.; Lach.;* MERC.; *Nit. ac.;* NUX v.; *Phos.;* SULPH.; SIL.; *Verat.; Zinc.*

Your leaders will be found under:

Belladonna, where they are worse from least jar; aversion to least motion; colic, worse from bending backwards. Staggers when rising from seat; headache; vertigo; pains in face, diarrhœa, metrorrhagia and cough worse from motion; cannot bear to stoop.

Bryonia, has general aggravation from least motion; walking, ascending, rising, stooping and a misstep aggravate conditions.

Colocynth, turning head, stooping and walking aggravates; rheumatism, pain in abdomen, and in eyes, are worse from motion.

Mercurius, pain in spine; joints; knee, palpitation, stitches and ulcers are worse.

Nux vom., ascending aggravates cough; on rising from seat vertigo and pain in right kidney are worse; turning in bed and walking aggravates brain and abdomen; staggers when walking.

9

Sulphur, headache; noise in ears; soreness between thighs, are worse from motion; walking aggravates head, sciatica, legs, burning soles (cramps in soles at every step); stooping makes head worse; ascending and rising from seat aggravate.

Silica, has general aggravation from even the slightest motion; stooping; rising and walking, aggravate complaints.

—

The following have *Particulars* aggravated from motion:

Apis, the headache, chill, stiffness and rheumatism are worse; stooping, walking, and least motion of hands, aggravate.

Arsenicum, headache, ovarian pains, constriction of chest, are worse; raising in bed aggravates headache; walking and ascending aggravate.

Arnica, headache, chills, chest, stomach, stiffness and soreness are worse.

Carbo veg., has difficult breathing on slightest motion; turning in bed and walking aggravate.

Digitalis, motion brings on angina pectoris; desire to urinate and defecate. Oppressed breathing and asthma when walking; palpitation and cyanosis from motion; cough worse from moving arms upward. Fears to move lest heart should stop.

Gelsemium, fears heart will stop unless he keeps constantly in motion; headache, eyelids, and cramps in legs, worse from motion.

Hepar, pain in back and limbs from walking up and down stairs; stooping and moving head aggravate headache.

Ipecac, slightest motion causes nausea; griping in intestines; sweat; cramps between scapulæ; cutting in intestines, and constriction of throat are worse.

Lachesis, has aversion to every kind of motion; walking aggravates vertigo and dyspnœa; headache, chest and suffocative attacks are worse.

Nitric acid, has vertigo; soreness in anus; stitches in vagina and sudden loss of breath when walking. Dyspnœa and palpitation on ascending; headache, chill and pain in abdomen, worse from motion.

Phosphorus, headache; dyspnœa; weakness in abdomen; exhaustion; pain in heel and staggers when walking; vertigo, cardialgia, palpitation, cough and involuntary stools, all aggravated from motion.

Veratrum alb., least motion aggravates nausea and vomiting. Rising aggravates the cough.

Headache, cutting in stomach, debility and dyspnœa are worse.

Zincum, slightest motion causes cutting pain from back into calves and feet; walking aggravates vertigo, headache, flatulent colic, burning anus, involuntary urine, and pain in knees and heel. Nausea, liver, chest and intercostal neuralgia are worse.

Aggravation During Afternoon.

Is covered by the following eighteen remedies:

Apis; BELL.; *Bry.; Coloc.; Dulc.; Dig.; Ign.;* LYC.; *Merc.; Nat. m.; Nit. ac.; Phos.;* PULS.; RHUS T.; SEP.; SIL.; THUJ.; ZINC.

Your leaders will be found under:

Belladonna, when worse from 3 P. M. to midnight.

Lycopodium, 3 or 4 and 4 to 8 P. M.

Pulsatilla, 3 to 6 P. M.; general aggravation in evening.

Rhus tox., fever worse at 2 P. M.; paroxysms appear at 5 P. M. in intermitent fever.

Sepia, has aggravation from 3 to 8 P. M.; fever, vertigo and pains worse.

Silica, has general evening and night aggravation; heat and thirst worse from 3 to 5 P. M.

Thuja, has chill at 5:30 P. M.; mucous stool at 6 P. M.; pressing in vertex worse.

Zincum, chill from 4 to 8 P. M.; cardialgia 3 to 4 P. M.; moroseness; vertigo, burning in eyes, sneezing, thirst, weakness and thoughts of death; sensitiveness to open air in afternoon.

Other Particulars that are aggravated in afternoon are found in the following:

Apis, has chill at 3 to 4 P. M.

Bryonia, headache; frequent urination worse 6 to 7 P. M.; sciatica and many complaints worse afternoon.

Colocynth, has aggravation from 4 to 9 P. M.

Digitalis, has 4 to 6 P. M. aggravation.

Dulcamara, general aggravation toward evening; pressing out headache, worse toward evening, on walking in open air; quarrelsome mood < P. M.

Ignatia, the pains gradually increase afternoon till evening; 4 P. M. aggravation.

Mercurius, chilly 5 to 6 P. M.; coldness in testicles in afternoon.

Natrum mur., has heat, chill, and cold feet, in afternoon.

Nitric acid, has cough, chill, vertigo, and incarcerated flatus, worse afternoon.

Phosphorus, has aggravation from 3 to 6 P. M.

Aggravation After Midnight.

Is covered by the following thirteen remedies:

ARS.; *Bry.; Calc. c.,* DROS.; *Gels.; Merc.;* NUX

v.; PHOS.; POD.; RHUS T.; *Sulph.;* SIL.; THUJ.

Your leaders will be:

Arsenicum, worse from 1 to 2 A. M.; anxiety; restlessness; diarrhœa; heat and coldness.

Drosera, has aggravation of nausea; cough; heat and cutting pains.

Nux vom., is worse from 3 to 4 A. M.; cough, renal colic and sweat, are worse.

Phosphorus, has aggravation of sweat, coryza and cough.

Podophyllum, has a diarrhœa with pain in abdomen at 3 A. M.; cramps in the intestines from 5 to 9 A. M.

Rhus tox., has general aggravation after midnight; restlessness, cramps and itching are worse.

Silica, has general aggravation after midnight. Chill 1 to 7 A. M.; wakens at 2 A. M.; sweat at 6 A. M.; diarrhœa from 6 to 8 A. M.

Thuja, has aggravation of chill; headache and rheumatism; pressing in vertex from 3 to 4 A. M.; chill at 3 A. M.

The following also have less marked aggravation after midnight:

Bryonia, < 3 to 6 A. M.

Calcarea carb., worse from 2 to 3 A. M.; sweat and cannot sleep after 3 A. M.

Gelsemium, has dreams; enuresis and leucorrhœa.

Mercurius, has thirst, ptyalism with nausea;
heat with violent thirst for cold drinks, worse
after midnight.

Sulphur, has aggravation at 4 and 5 A. M.;
sweat after waking from 6 to 7 A. M.; cough
until 2 A. M.

Aggravation After Sleep.

Is found in the following fourteen remedies:

*Acon.; Arn.; Ars.; Apis; Carbo v.; Caust.;
Hep.;* LACH.; *Lyco.; Phos.; Phos. ac.; Puls.;
Rhus;* SULPH.

Your leaders under this rubric will be:

Lachesis, where there is general aggravation
after sleep and where complaints come on during
sleep.

Sulphur, starts and screams after sleep;
wakens frightened; diarrhœa after sleep.

The following have aggravation after sleep
in the second degree:

Aconite, on going to sleep fever becomes intolerable; starts from nightmare.

Apis, sleeps into <; wakes weary. Starts
from sleep suddenly with great anxiety.

Arnica, paralyzed on right side; < after a
long sleep; unrefreshed by sleep.

Arsenicum, starts from sleep and is weary after sleep.

Carbo veg., has aggravation of coldness of feet and legs after sleep.

Causticum, is worse on awaking; must sit up; cramps in heels after sleep.

Hepar, fright during and suffocation after sleep.

Lycopodium, is hungry and unrefreshed; cross; kicks and scolds after sleep.

Phosphoric acid, has sad thoughts; dry heat and hunger after sleep.

Phosphorus, is anxious and unrefreshed.

Pulsatilla, has indigestion and is languid and unrefreshed after sleep.

Rhus tox., is anxious, weak, restless, trembling, and it seems as if he had not slept.

Aggravation from Pressure.

Is found in the following twelve remedies:

Ars.; APIS; *Carbo v.;* HEP.; LACH.; LYC.; *Merc.; Nat. m.; Nit. ac.; Nux;* SIL.; STAPH.

Your leaders will be:

Apis, is sensitive to light touch, cannot bear the sheet to touch skin; every hair is painful; child stiffens when touched.

Hepar, has dread of contact and extreme sensitiveness; scalp, eye, renal region, muscles of neck and external throat are aggravated from pressure.

Lachesis, is worse from slightest touch; pressure produces black and blue marks; pressure on larynx causes cough; throat and abdomen sensitive. (Sometimes firm pressure > when light touch is not tolerated.)

Lycopodium, is sensitive to pressure in all soft parts; tight clothes and weight of clothes aggravate; liver especially sensitive.

Silica, cannot tolerate pressure below floating ribs; scalp and pit of stomach worse from pressure; parts on which he lies go to sleep. Touch aggravates drawing in head, toothache, eye, liver, vagina, and pain in elbows.

Staphisagria, neuralgia of scalp, ovary and ulcers, are worse from pressure; touch aggravates drawing in head, toothache, ulcers and knee-joint.

———

Particulars under following are aggravated from pressure in second degree:

Arsenicum, has scalp, stomach and abdominal symptoms aggravated from pressure.

Carbo veg., the scalp, liver and perineum are aggravated.

Mercurius, has aggravation of head, teeth,

gums, stomach, liver, bladder, spine, ulcers and bone pains.

Natrum mur., must loosen clothing; touching hair causes it to fall out; nose, jaw, teeth, epigastrium and spine are aggravated.

Nitric acid, condylomata bleed when touched; eruption, iritis, teeth, abdomen, anus and ulcer are worse from touch.

Nux vom., tight clothing aggravates soreness over liver; touching with the hand brings on spasm; stomach, liver, scalp and abdomen are aggravated by pressure.

Relief from Pressure.

Is found in the following ten remedies:

Apis; BRY.; CHINA; COLOC.; DROS.; *Dulc.;* *Graph.;* PULS.; *Rhus;* SIL.

Your leaders for this amelioration will be:

Bryonia, has general relief from pressure.

China, has a drawing headache and pressure from middle of sternum, which is relieved; pressure in region of liver relieved by bending body forward.

Colocynth, is relieved by firm, hard, pressure.

Drosera, holds chest firmly when coughing or sneezing; pains in face, stomach, and stitches in chest relieved by pressure.

Pulsatilla, hard rubbing relieves; headache, left chest, pains in arm and throbbing in arteries, relieved by pressure.

Silica, while many of the pains are *worse* from touch and pressure the headache is *relieved* by hard pressure or by tying the head tightly.

The following *particulars* are relieved by pressure:

Apis, has a headache relieved by pressure while all other symptoms are worse.

Dulcamara, the pains in chest and stitches in back are relieved.

Graphites, has a colic relieved by pressure, although the liver and abdomen are worse from tight clothing and pressure.

Rhus tox., has a sciatica relieved by rubbing; pain in back, right nates, crest of left ilium, hip and legs are relieved.

Thirst.

The following twenty-one remedies have THIRST in the first or second degree:

ACON.; *Arn.;* ARS.; *Bell.;* BRY.; CALC. C.; CHAM.; CHINA; DIG.; *Hyos.; Lach.;* MERC.; *Nux v.;* NAT. M.; *Nit. ac.;* PHOS.; *Podo.;* RHUS; SULPH.; SIL.; VERAT.

This rubric is common to many disease conditions and to many remedies. If there is nothing to account for the thirst it is an important symptom, but if the patient is running a high temperature, or is working in the heat, or has a disease like diabetes it would be a common thing for him to be thirsty, and under such circumstances your symptom of thirst would have no place in your symptom picture.

Your leaders for general and particular thirst symptoms will be:

Aconite, has a burning, unquenchable thirst and desires bitter drinks, wine, brandy and beer.

Arsenicum, wants cold water a little and often; burning, unquenchable, thirst during sweat; desires acids, coffee, milk, wine, beer and brandy.

Bryonia, has a great thirst with internal heat; wants large drinks at long intervals; warm drinks relieve.

Calcarea carb., has a thirst which drinking does not relieve, worse at night; desires cold drinks and acids.

Chamomilla, has thirst for cold water and weakness and nausea after drinking coffee; toothache relieved by hot water; desires acids.

China, has thirst before or after chill and during sweat; wants to drink little and often.

Digitalis, has a continuous thirst with dry lips; desires sour and bitter drinks.

Mercurius, has a moist tongue with burning thirst for cold drinks.

Natrum mur., has a constant thirst without desire to drink, worse in the evening; longing for bitter, sour things and for milk, with aversion to coffee.

Phosphorus, wants very cold drinks; his stomach is relieved by them until they become warm, when they are vomited. Desire for refreshing drinks, with aversion to boiled milk, coffee and tea.

Rhus tox., has a dry throat at night and wants only cold drinks.

Silica, has want of appetite but excessive thirst; desires cold drinks.

Sulphur, drinks much and eats little; violent thirst for ale and beer.

Veratrum alb., wants everything ice cold, little and often; desires cold drinks.

—

The following remedies will be of use when their particular thirst is present:

Arnica, has a thirst for cold water without fever; constant desire for vinegar.

Belladonna, great thirst, but drinking suffocates; desires lemonade.

Hyoscyamus, has a dread of water; unquenchable thirst with inability to swallow.

Lachesis, constant thirst, but is afraid to drink; disgust for drink.

Nux vom., has thirst during chill; in morning; desire for beer and brandy.

Nitric acid, violent thirst in the morning.

Podophyllum, great thirst for large quantities of cold water. Desires sour things.

Aggravation From Eating and After Eating.

Is found in the following twenty-seven remedies, either in the first or second degree:

Ars.; *Ant. t.; Bell.;* Bry.; *Cham.;* Calc. c.; *China; Carbo v.;* Caust.; Coloc.; *Graph.;* *Hyos.;* Lach.; Lyc.; Nux v.; Nat. m.; *Nit. ac.;* Phos.; Phos. ac.; Puls.; *Podo.; Rhus t.;* Sulph.; Sep.; Sil.; *Thuj.;* Zinc.

Your leaders under this rubric will be:

Arsenicum, feels better on an empty stomach; bitter taste, nausea, painless stools and chill are worse after eating.

Bryonia, has many symptoms directly after dinner; weight and pressure in stomach after eating; complains from eating oysters, old sausage, old cheese, salads, cabbage and potatoes, fresh, green vegetables. Pertussis worse after eating.

Calcarea carb., nausea and pressure in stomach after eating. Toothache, cough, heart symptoms, stool and heat worse from eating.

Causticum, complaints from eating bread, fat and fresh meat.

Colocynth, has diarrhœa from least food or drink; colic from potatoes; griping and flatulency after eating; pains worse from eating or drinking.

Lachesis, has vertigo; languor; drowsiness; dyspnœa; flashes of heat; pressing in stomach; diarrhœa after eating or made worse by eating.

Lycopodium, fills up after a few mouthfuls; drowsiness; pressure in stomach and liver; spitting up food after eating; bad effects from onions, oysters and rye bread.

Nux vom., is so sleepy after eating; must loosen clothing after; hypochondriacal mood, sour taste, pressure and pyrosis, after eating; also cough is worse.

Natrum mur., always feels better on empty stomach; sweat on face, while eating; nausea, palpitation and acidity after eating.

Phosphorus, has pains which begin while eating and last until he stops; desires cold food and drink; nausea, belching and fulness of stomach after eating.

Pulsatilla, is useful in bad effects from pastry, rich foods, fats, onions and buckwheat.

Sulphur, drinks much and eats little; complaints aggravated from eating even a little; milk disagrees.

Sepia, has pains aggravated immediately after eating; aggravation from bread, milk, fats and acids.

Silica, has chilliness on back and icy cold feet after eating in evening; sour eructations, fulness in stomach; waterbrash and vomiting large amounts of water after eating. Aversion to mother's milk; vomiting whenever taking it.

Zincum, has heartburn from eating sugar; worse from wine and milk.

Worse after eating is given in the second degree in the following remedies:

Antimonium tart., has somewhat of relief of pressure in stomach after eating; still eating sour food brings on attack of asthma.

Belladonna, has pressure in stomach and putrid taste in mouth after eating.

Chamomilla, heat and sweat of face during and after; vertigo, nausea and abdomen puffed up after eating.

China, is drowsy, and uneasy after eating; headache and fulness in stomach after.

Carbo veg., dreads to eat because of pain; headache, acid mouth, heaviness, fulness, hot eructations, and burning in stomach, after eating; feels as if abdomen would burst after meals; butter, fats, fish and pastry disagree.

Graphites, has disgust for and nausea from sweet things; hot things disagree.

Hyoscyamus, has hiccough with spasms and rumbling after eating.

Nitric acid, has bitter taste; heavy weight in stomach, debility, heat and palpitation after eating; food causes acidity; fat food causes nausea and acidity.

Phosphoric acid, has pressing in stomach and bitter eructations after eating; diarrhœa from acids and sour foods.

Podophyllum, has a craving appetite after eating; nausea and vomiting of food one hour after eating; diarrhœa and sour hot eructations after eating.

Rhus tox., sleepiness, fulness in stomach and giddiness after eating.

Thuja, for the bad effects of beer, fat, acid, sweets, tobacco, tea, wine and onions.

—

The character of the pain is a symptom always brought out by the patient; under

Burning Pains.

We find the following twenty-eight remedies:

Acon.; *Arn.;* Ars.; *Apis;* Bell.; Bry.; *China;*

10

Carbo v., Caust.; Coloc.; Dulc.; Dros.; Graph.; Ign.; Lach.; Lyc.; MERC.; NAT. M.; NIT. AC.; NUX V.; PHOS.; PHOS. AC.; PULS.; RHUS; SULPH.; SEP.; SIL.; *Zinc.*

Your leaders for this rubric will be:

Aconite, where there is burning in internal parts; of the lips and tongue.

Arsenicum, has burning pains relieved by heat; through the veins; head, eyes, nose, ulcers, mucous membrane, liver, ovaries, back, spine and joints burn.

Belladonna, has burning in eyes, nose, stomach, throat, chest and ovary.

Bryonia, the head, eyes, ribs, liver, abdomen, stool, urine and chest have burning.

Graphites, has old scars that burn; spot on vertex, eyes, tongue, stomach, left hypochondrium, through abdomen, vagina, soles of feet and hands, burn or have pains burning in character.

Mercurius, has general stinging and burning pains relieved by heat; burning internally; burning after scratching.

Natrum mur., has burning pains aggravated by heat of sun and of stove; relieved by washing in cold water and by open air; burning pains in vertex, eyes, ears, nose, throat, stomach, bowels, urethra, vagina, hands and feet.

Nitric acid, general burning, stinging and sticking pains.

Nux vomica, has internal burning; burning pains in head; throat, stomach, abdomen, anus, back, bladder and chest.

Phosphorus, has general burning pains in head, brain, chest and under sternum in particular.

Phosphoric acid, burning pains worse lower half of the body; general burning, liver, throat and chest in particular.

Pulsatilla, has burning in eyes, throat, bladder, urethra, feet, chest and heart.

Rhus tox., has burning, stinging and drawing pains worse on left side.

Sulphur, has burning in general, with burning heat; burning in skin of whole body and in parts on which he lies; burning pains in vertex, forehead, palms, eyes, lids, nostrils, face, throat, of eczema, fauces, pharynx, stomach, abdomen, urethra, anus, in hæmorrhoids, between scapulæ, hands, balls and tips of fingers, knee, feet (particularly at night), soles, corns and chilblains.

Sepia, has internal burning with relief in open air; feet and palms burn. Hands hot and feet cold or vice versa.

Silica, has general burning, stinging pains; burning in soles of feet and in ulcers.

Zincum, has burning pains · in back, whole length of spine, left arm, right wrist and ball of hand, left hip, soles, skin and ulcers.

———

Those burning pains not covered by the above list will be found under:

Arnica, has burning pains in brain, eyes, lips, throat,. stomach, chest, heart and feet.

Apis, has general burning, stinging pains.

China, has burning of one hand while the other is icy cold; burning of the skin, and in ulcers.

Carbo veg., general burning as from coals of fire, without thirst, and better from cold.

Causticum, general burning pains; burning in spots as from ball of fire.

Colocynth, has burning in right side of forehead; eyelids, face, tongue, back, anus, urethra (during stool), right ovary and sciatic nerve.

Dulcamara, burning in forehead, epigastrium, anus, rectum, meatus, feet, gums and back.

Drosera, burning deep in throat and center of chest.

Ignatia, has burning redness of one ear and cheek; burning heat in vagina and feet; pain in head, eyes, epigastrium, stomach, urethra and heels.

Lachesis, has burning, stinging pains in top

of head, eyes, mouth, rectum, ovary, wrists, stomach, from hip to foot, throat, hands and soles.

Lycopodium, has one foot burning hot, the other cold; burning in blisters on tongue; thumb and third finger of left hand; pain in stomach, rectum, lower limbs and ankles; and of wounds.

Cutting Pains.

Are covered by the following seventeen remedies:

Arn.; Bell.; Calc. c.; *Chin.;* Coloc.; Dros.; Hyos.; Lyc.; Merc.; Nux v.; Nat. m.; Puls.; Sulph.; Sil.; *Staph.;* Verat.; Zinc.

Your leaders will be found in:

Belladonna, where the cutting pains are in head (right side), face, stomach, abdomen, uterus and in the muscles.

Calcarea carb., where there are cutting pains from within outward; pains in chest; stomach, back and liver.

Colocynth, cutting as from knives in bowels; pain in forehead, left temple, eyes, ears, stomach, abdomen and chest.

Drosera, cutting pains mostly in right side; in calves of legs.

Hyoscyamus, cutting in abdomen, chest and joints.

Lycopodium, has cutting in bladder, rectum, abdomen, liver, chest, scalp and penis.

Mercurius, has dull, cutting, pressive and stitching pains; cutting from stomach to genitals; pains in eyes, abdomen and intestines.

Nux vomica, has shooting, cutting pains about navel.

Natrum mur., has pains in head, abdomen, urethra, chest and back.

Pulsatilla, cutting in bowels, throat, abdomen, limbs, liver, chest, back and in abscesses.

Silica, cutting pains in nerves; in right lung, testes, breast, shoulders, knee, stomach, rectum and about navel.

Sulphur, has cutting, burning pains in eyelids and urethra; cutting in abdomen, loins and sacrum, vesical region, chest, about heart and in great toe.

Veratrum alb., cutting, griping colic; pain in left chest.

Zincum, in small of back during menses; cross umbilical region; pain in right eye and ear, nose, rectum, anus, kidney and urethra.

—

Cutting pains are also found in:

Arnica, has cutting like knives in kidney; pain in teeth, epigastrium and liver.

China, has cutting pains which shoot through abdomen in all directions before the passage of flatus; cutting in spleen as if it was hardened.

Staphisagria, for injuries caused by sharp cutting instruments; pain over crural nerve; teeth and abdomen; pains in stitches after operations.

Sore Pains.

Are covered by the following twelve remedies: ARN.; BELL.; CHINA; DROS.; HEP.; NUX V.; NAT. M.; *Phos.;* RHUS T.; SULPH.; SIL.; ZINC.

Your leaders will be found under:

Arnica, for bad effects of bruises and sprains; pain is sore as if bruised in head; brain, throat and stomach; general character of pains *sore.*

Belladonna, has soreness and rawness; pains in eyelids, throat to ears, abdomen and back.

China, has sore pains worse from light touch but relieved by hard pressure; sore all over in the joints, bones, periosteum, as if they had been sprained.

Drosera, soreness in temples and in skin of right temple; bruised feeling in the larynx, back and ankle.

Hepar, soreness in urethra, in genitals, scrotum, in folds between scrotum and thighs, chest and in all the limbs; bruised feeling in anterior muscles of thighs.

Nux vomica, has soreness all over; great tenderness of abdomen; soreness in liver, stomach, abdomen, across pubis, chest and shoulder-joint;

bruised sensation of brain, in small of back, neck of uterus, low down in abdomen; in back and in limbs.

Natrum mur., soreness left side of nose; nostrils; upper arm; epigastrium; chest; tarsal joints; liver; vulva; vagina; larynx and trachea and between the toes.

Phosphorus, bruised feeling in bones; soreness and rawness; nose, mouth, chest, lungs, larynx and bronchi are sore.

Rhus tox., has soreness and stiffness; soreness in head, nostrils, tongue, abdomen, of navel, in muscles of abdomen, back, vagina, chest and left side of lumbar region; bruised feeling in head, throat and limbs.

Sulphur, sore pain in left eye, in oral commissures, and in whole abdomen; bruised feeling and pain in abdomen, back, coccyx, left shoulder, left hip, thighs, in sciatic region and lower extremities.

Silica, the eyeballs are stiff and sore; internal soreness; sore pain in bones, chest, lungs and head.

Zincum, has soreness in head, vertex, scalp and hair; pterygium; right upper lid; outer canthus; in nose, teeth, tongue, upper chest and left hypochondrium; rectum, anus, left kidney, urethra;

as if beaten in the pectoral muscles; chest; outer muscles of thigh and in pimples.

Throbbing Pains.

Are covered by the following fourteen remedies:

ACON.; *Bell.; Bry.; Cham.;* CALC. C.; *Ign.; Nit. ac.;* PHOS.; *Puls.; Rhus t.; Sulph.;* SEP.; *Sil.; Staph.*

Your leaders will be found under:

Aconite, where there is throbbing in temples and left side of head.

Calcarea carb., throbbing in ulcers; pain in vertex and forehead, worse from motion.

Phosphorus, throbbing forehead, temples, teeth, heart, extending to throat, back and neck.

Pulsatilla, throbbing in brain, head, forehead, teeth, ear and soles of feet.

Sepia, has throbbing in temple, forehead, cerebellum and teeth.

———

When the above do not cover your case look to the following:

Belladonna, has throbbing in carotids, in brain, teeth, stomach, ovary and breasts. While this remedy is given in routine practice for throbbing pains it does not have this symptom in as marked degree as the remedies given above. It will only cure throbbing pains when the rest of the symptoms agree.

Bryonia, has throbbing throughout the body; pain in vertex.

Chamomilla, has a throbbing in one-half of the brain and in the back part of throat.

Ignatia, has throbbing pain in right forehead, temples and occiput.

Nitric acid, has throbbing pain in left side of head; ears, nape of neck, small of back, teeth and stomach.

Rhus tox., throbbing in pit of stomach; in temples and from jaws and teeth into temples; in left shoulder and forehead.

Silica, has throbbing pain in forehead and up nito head; in eyes, in teeth and in limbs; sacral region; in forehead and vertex with chilliness.

Staphisagria, has throbbing in temples and from tooth to eye.

Sulphur, throbbing pain in left side of occiput; in hand, teeth, gums, rectum and anus.

Cramping Pains.

Are covered by the following ten remedies:

Bell.; Calc. c.; Dig.; Nat. m.; Phos.; Phos. ac.; Puls.; *Sulph.; Staph.; Zinc.*

Your leaders will be:

Phosphoric acid, where there are cramps in joints; upper arm; wrist; chest; stomach; diaphragm and abdomen.

Pulsatilla, cramping pain in stomach, through chest; in right leg from knee to groin; in legs, abdomen, and in pit of stomach.

———

The following have crampy pains in second degree:

Belladonna, has cramps in jaws; the cramping pain in abdomen and stomach is relieved by lying at an angle of 45 degrees, and is aggravated by bending back; cramps in uterus and muscles are found under this remedy.

Calcarea carb., has cramps in the hands and forearms, feet and legs, crampy pains in hypochondria and in stomach, with palpitation.

Digitalis, has cramps in chest, abdomen and bladder.

Natrum mur., has cramping pains in abdomen at menses; crampy colic pains that resemble labor pains, aggravated after stool and relieved by passing flatus; pains in arms, hands, fingers, thumbs, legs, calves and feet.

Phosphorus, has crampy pains in testes, stomach, rectum, calves, between scapulæ, and in left side of head.

Staphisagria, has crampy pains in abdomen, right knee joint, and first joints of fingers.

Sulphur, has crampy pains in stomach, chest;